Praise for

SEX MATTERS

"McGregor is to be commended for showing how medicine has long skewed male and harmed women. Especially spot-on are the chapters on implicit bias, treatment of women of color, and issues affecting trans individuals. The author concludes with to-do lists, questions women can ask their providers, and suggestions for advocacy roles to raise awareness of the issues. Good ammunition for mandating sex- and gender-based differences in health professional education, research, and practice."

—*Kirkus Reviews*

"This book is addictive! You will not be able to put it down until you have read it from cover to cover and then want to start all over again. The sheer wealth of information is an eye-opener for the intelligent lay person and a great source of up-to-date information for healthcare workers."

—Marek Glezerman, MD, Immediate Past-President,
International Society for Gender Medicine

"Alyson McGregor is a persuasive and intelligent advocate for the unique healthcare needs of women. The two sexes are significantly different in all the tissues of the body—even to the way the same genes are expressed. An expert in emergency medical care, her deep and informed knowledge of the way disease presents itself in women ensures their prompt and accurate diagnosis and treatment. She is a powerful force in gender-specific health care."

—Marianne J. Legato, MD, PhD (hon. c.), FACP,
Emerita Professor of Clinical Medicine,
Columbia University

"Dr. Alyson McGregor sounds the alarm for the state of women's health in this country. Her excellent, evidence-based book reveals that women's health is still in its infancy and needs significant research to ensure that women are receiving the best possible medical care. The fact that most drugs that were approved in this country did not even have enough women included in the studies that got them approved to know if the effects in women were the same as in men is just one of many concerning findings. Her book shows that there is much work to do in this area (much more even than we thought) and that we can count on this call to action to spur us onward! This book will be appreciated by medical and lay people alike, given its excellent readability. I am thrilled that this book is out there to provide benchmarks and goals so that we can ultimately transform women's health."

—Judy Regensteiner, MD, Director of the Center for Women's Health Research at the University of Colorado

"Dr. McGregor makes a clear and compelling case that women, particularly women of color, in the United States time after time receive inadequate or even harmful medical care. Dr. McGregor also explains how cultural stereotypes about women are frequently used by physicians to justify a dismissive approach to women's symptoms, even when these symptoms herald conditions with potentially dire outcomes. Taking it one step further, Dr. McGregor provides the reader with suggestions on how to cut through a physician's ability to dismiss her symptoms, encouraging her to find another provider if necessary."

—Molly Carnes, MD, MS, Virginia Valian Professor, Departments of Medicine, Psychiatry, and Industrial and Systems Engineering, Director, Center for Women's Health Research, Codirector, Women in Science and Engineering Leadership Institute (WISELI), University of Wisconsin-Madison

"I have worked with Dr. Alyson McGregor as a national leader in the area of sex and gender in medicine and health care—I commend her on this book."

—C. Noel Bairey Merz, MD, Director, Barbra Streisand Women's Heart Center, Cedars-Sinai

SEX MATTERS

SEX MATTERS

MATTERS

How male-centric medicine
endangers women's health and
what we can do about it

DR ALYSON J. MCGREGOR

Quercus

First published in the USA by Hachette Go, an imprint of Perseus Books, LLC,
a subsidiary of Hachette Book Group, Inc. New York.

First published in hardback Great Britain in 2020 by Quercus Editions Ltd

This paperback edition published in 2021 by

Quercus Editions Ltd
Carmelite House
50 Victoria Embankment
London EC4Y 0DZ

An Hachette UK company

Copyright © 2020 by Alyson J. McGregor, MD

The moral right of Alyson J. McGregor to be
identified as the author of this work has been
asserted in accordance with the
Copyright, Designs and Patents Act, 1988.

All rights reserved. No part of this publication
may be reproduced or transmitted in any form
or by any means, electronic or mechanical,
including photocopy, recording, or any
information storage and retrieval system,
without permission in writing from the publisher.

A CIP catalogue record for this book is available
from the British Library

ISBN 978 1 52940 592 7

Quercus Editions Ltd hereby exclude all liability to the extent permitted by law for any errors
or omissions in this book and for any loss, damage or expense (whether direct or indirect)
suffered by a third party relying on any information contained in this book.

Note: The information in this book is true and complete to the best of our
knowledge. This book is intended only as an informative guide for those wishing
to know more about health issues. In no way is this book intended to replace,
countermand, or conflict with the advice given to you by your own doctor,
and we strongly recommend you follow his or her advice. Information in
this book is general and is offered with no guarantees on the part of the authors
or Quercus Editions Ltd. The authors and publisher disclaim all liability in connection
with the use of this book. The names and identifying details of people associated
with events described in this book have been changed. Any similarity to actual
persons is coincidental.

10 9 8 7 6 5 4 3

Printed and bound in Great Britain by Clays Ltd, Elcograf S.p.A.

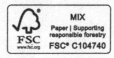

Papers used by Quercus are from well-managed forests and other responsible sources.

THIS BOOK IS DEDICATED TO

All the women I have had the pleasure to care for,
who taught me about their illnesses and insight.

All the women whose struggles I have witnessed
through our medical system, through everything
from lack of understanding, to questioning self-
reflection, to endless testing that leaves them feeling
dismissed, they have persevered.

AND ALSO TO

My mother and sister, with immense love and
gratitude. As I studied medicine, I watched the
two of you navigate our medical system from the
outside; you helped me see the full circle.

CONTENTS

Contents

PART THREE

WHERE WE'RE HEADED— AND WHAT YOU CAN DO

171

FOREWORD

Recently, I delivered a presentation on sex and gender in medicine at a top-tier medical school in the U.S. After the assembly concluded, a colleague asked me if I'd like to take a tour of the facility. Of course, I happily agreed. I get excited whenever I get to see firsthand the advances we're making in medical education.

Great strides were certainly being made here. The students at this institution had access to top-notch new technologies, beautiful work spaces, and world-class instructors. We toured the lecture halls, the anatomy lab, the student lounge, and the study areas.

"Want to see the sim lab?" my colleague asked.

"Absolutely!" The simulation laboratory, or "sim lab" for short, is where students get to practice clinical skills, procedures, teamwork, and communication skills on high-tech mannequins designed to look and feel like real human bodies. (We've come a long way from the days of the Edinburgh body snatchers!) Sim labs have evolved drastically in recent years, becoming more lifelike and detailed than ever, and I was excited to take in this latest iteration.

When we opened the door to the lab, I gasped aloud.

Bodies lay on the metal tables in neat rows. Some were opened to reveal organs and tissues, others sported bruises, contusions, or deep penetration wounds meant to simulate everything from car accidents to stabbings. But it wasn't the graphic scene that startled me; I see all that and more on a daily basis in the emergency department where I work.

No, what shocked me was that *every one of the sim bodies in that room was white and male.* There were no female bodies. There was no diversity in skin tone, or even body shape. The only "female" body was a male sim wearing a blonde wig. A plastic fetus and placenta were lying next to it on the table.

My colleague looked sick. "I hadn't been in here yet," she admitted. "I had no idea."

I nodded. Even in the most "advanced" medical institutions, we are still locked into a mode of male centricity.

You may be thinking, "Why does it matter? Who cares about the sex of the sim bodies in a medical school?"

The answer is, we *all* should care.

Sim labs like this one are part of a larger system of medical education that treats the white, male norm as the *only* norm. Students are trained to look for male patterns of disease, trauma, and pain on male bodies, and solve problems according to research and testing conducted using mostly male models. This system ultimately creates doctors who ascribe to the false belief that, aside from their sex organs, men and women are biologically identical. And this belief is hurting women the world over.

I wrote this book to increase awareness about the overwhelming male centricity of our medical system and inspire activism on a grass-roots level among women who are tired of experiencing substandard outcomes and biased treatment in medical care situations. While I am a physician practicing in the United States, I know that this issue is not confined to the American health system. In the medical community, information and research are shared globally. And as long as our standards for research, testing, and education allow for male-focused and male-centric practices to abide, our tools for providing care to women will be fundamentally flawed.

As you'll learn in this book, women are biologically different from men from their DNA on up. We have different internal mechanisms that affect the outward expressions of disease, from differences in metabolic processes and pathways to sex-specific response to treatments. We know this because new technology has provided us with access to more and better information about women's bodies than ever before. And because we know the difference now, it is no longer acceptable for women in any part of the world, in any medical culture or system, to receive care that doesn't take their unique bodies into account.

By picking up this book, you have become part of the solution. The pathways to self-education, advocacy, and grass-roots change I've laid out in the book are transferrable to women in any medical system, in every part of the world. While the details of how we receive care may be different depending on where we live, the foundational information about how women's bodies differ from men's is universal.

Thank you for taking this journey with me.

Yours in health,
Alyson J. McGregor, MD, MA, FACEP
March 2020, Providence, Rhode Island, U.S.A.

INTRODUCTION

As an undergraduate in the University of New Hampshire's premed program, I took only one elective that wasn't directly related to my major (or, at least, I thought at the time that it wasn't related). That course was women's studies. I loved circling up with other women to talk about the history of women in society and the gender-related issues we faced both individually and collectively. It was illuminating and truly inspiring. When the class ended, and our spirited discussions were replaced in my schedule by yet another biology lab, I felt like a bit of the spark had gone out of my collegiate life.

I didn't know it at the time, but that course—and the questions about sex, gender, and the female experience it sparked in me—would have a profound influence on the trajectory of my career.

When I finished medical school at the Boston University School of Medicine, I applied for a residency at Brown University in my hometown of Providence, Rhode Island. When my residency ended, I wanted to stay on and work there. Because Brown is an academic institution, I needed to choose a research focus in order to apply for a long-term position. When I sat down and thought about it, the only path I wanted to take was one that would improve the lives and health of women. I wanted to know about women's bodies and how those bodies affected (and were affected by) modern medicine—in particular, emergency medicine.

At the time, sex and gender research didn't even exist. My choice to pursue a specialty in women's health felt like a nod to my feminist beliefs and personal philosophy, a way to keep feeding my passion for women's issues.

I had no idea just how deep an ocean I was diving into or how many challenges I would face in bringing women's unique health concerns into the medical mainstream.

When I mentioned to my advisors that I'd like to explore fields related to women's health, the immediate reaction was, "Oh. You want to do OB/GYN."

"No," I'd reply. "I want to study women's health holistically. As in, the overall health of women."

No one seemed to know what I meant. That was my first clue about what was really happening in our medical establishment.

As I discovered, and as I'll share in this book, there is far more to "women's health" than pelvic exams and mammography. Women are different from men in every way, from their DNA on up. The medical practice of differentiating women from men according to their reproductive organs alone is both reductionist and, as it turns out, hugely problematic—but the male-centric model of medicine is so pervasive in our healthcare systems, procedures, and philosophy that many don't even realize it exists. Most people simply assume that women's differences are already being taken into account—yet nothing could be further from the truth.

My research on and passion for this issue has placed me at the forefront of a medical revolution. As a researcher, educator, speaker, and physician, I—and my colleagues in this cutting-edge field—are tasked with integrating emerging information about women's health into the mainstream medical culture. We are advocates for women and their unique bodies in a system that has largely ignored them, marginalized them, and minimized them. We are women (and a few good men) taking a stand for women in a way that has never been done before.

Awareness Is the First Step to Change

As an internationally-recognized expert on sex and gender medicine, I have made researching and bringing awareness to health disparities between men and women across all areas of medicine my life's work. In addition to my "day job" seeing patients in the emergency department of an urban trauma center—and dealing with everything from colds to car accidents, headaches to heart attacks, and broken bones to overdoses—I wear a few other hats: I'm the division director for the first program in sex and gender emergency medicine at the Alpert Medical School of Brown University and a cofounder of the Sex and Gender Women's Health Collaborative. I am also a sought-after visiting professor and Grand Rounds speaker at medical institutions across the country, and I'm a keynote speaker for community advocacy groups, including the Laura Bush Institute for Women's Health, the Barbra Streisand Women's Heart Center, the National Aeronautics and Space Administration, the Society for Women's Health Research, the Organization for the Study of Sex Differences, and the Office of Women in Medicine and Science at Brown University, among others. I've written or cowritten over seventy peer-reviewed publications in scientific journals on the topic of sex and gender, and I'm the lead editor for the medical textbook *Sex and Gender in Acute Care Medicine*.

While much of my work is accomplished within the medical community itself—through educating medical students and professionals, advocating for changes in research guidelines and pharmaceutical prescribing standards, and conducting research on sex and gender issues—changing the system from within is only half the battle. The other half is educating the women whose lives and health are being impacted by that system every single day. My TEDx talk, "Why Medicine Often Has Dangerous Side Effects for Women," was intended to open the eyes of women around the world to the issues discussed in this book.

Every time I talk about sex and gender issues in medicine, I hear stories from women about how the system has ignored, minimized, or outright failed them. This failure of care may not be intentional on the part of women's doctors and providers—but neither is it acceptable.

How to Use This Book

While this book contains facts and observations that you may find revelatory or even shocking, my intention is for it to serve as far more than an exposé.

Ultimately, information is more useful when it's actionable. It's not enough for us to merely observe the scope of the problems women face in our modern medical system or even to voice our feelings of anger and betrayal at what we see; we need to always be asking, "What can we *do* about this?"

This book is intended to be both informative and prescriptive. By the time you turn the last page, I hope that you will understand not only how male-centric medicine affects women in both broad and specific terms but also exactly what steps you, personally, can take right now to begin to reduce your personal risk factors and make grassroots changes in your local medical community.

In Part I of this book, we will look at the broad picture of male-centric medicine: how it came to be, how it works in practice, and how its lack of recognition of women's physiological differences is jeopardizing the health of women around the world.

In Part II, we will look at specific disease patterns and areas of health that impact millions of women globally—including heart attacks, strokes, pain disorders, pain management, and pharmaceuticals. We'll also look at the role of women's hormones and biochemistry in various areas of health, as well as at how issues and biases related to gender, race, ethnicity, and religion affect medical treatment and outcomes both subtly and explicitly.

In Part III, I'll write you a prescription for action! We will look at how the landscape of medicine is changing for the better and how you can tap into existing resources to take a more active role in your own health care. In Chapter 10, I'll share specific questions you can ask your providers to help you get the answers you need, as well as resources to assist you in your own research.

By picking up this book, you have become part of a movement for change. You have chosen to educate yourself about the realities of how modern medicine treats women and their bodies. Throughout this book, I will give you tools to translate your new awareness into advocacy—for yourself and for other women like you.

As a patient and as a woman, you have a voice—and your voice matters. This book will equip you to use your voice effectively in a medical setting. You'll learn what questions to ask, what pitfalls to look out for, what tests to request or avoid, and what resources to employ so that you can receive the quality of care you need and deserve. Effectively, you will become a more equal partner in your own health care.

ON THE NEXT PAGE, you will begin your journey into the discovery of women's health as it stands in our current medical system. You will learn things that will surprise you and many that may distress you. But in the end, I hope that you will find in these pages a feeling of empowerment and the knowledge you need to become a voice for your own health and the health of women everywhere.

Are you ready to get started?

PART ONE

HOW WE
GOT HERE

chapter one

MODERN MEDICINE *IS* MALE-CENTRIC MEDICINE

I'LL NEVER FORGET THE DAY that a thirty-two-year-old woman almost walked out of my emergency department while having a heart attack.

In emergency medicine, there are many algorithms by which we evaluate risk factors and stratify incoming patients. Not everyone who walks through the doors of the emergency department is on death's door, so we treat the most urgent cases first. For example, someone who's asphyxiating or suffering from a stab wound will be regarded as a higher priority than someone suffering from nonspecific pain or who "just doesn't feel quite right."

This risk assessment makes sense theoretically and works fairly well in practice too. But once the obvious cases have been dealt with, we're navigating a large gray area. Unfortunately, the subtle (and often subjective) strata by which we prioritize patients who don't appear to be at immediate risk are far from perfect—particularly when those patients are women.

Women are different from men in more ways than merely the obvious—and nowhere is this more apparent than in the halls of the hospital where I work and teach every day.

For example, the research upon which our stratification procedures are based cites things like the "estrogen-protective effect" (meaning, the way in which blood estrogen levels appear to reduce or modify traditional risk factors like oxidative stress, arrhythmia, and fibrosis in premenopausal women) and the supposedly low statistical likelihood of premenopausal women presenting with acute heart conditions. In other words, even if a young woman were to come into the ED and say, "I think I'm having a heart attack," unless she displayed blatant and very specific symptoms, most doctors would immediately look for another explanation.

Julie, the young woman I met that day, had visited her primary care doctor several times prior to coming to the emergency department and had also seen at least two other physicians in the previous forty-eight hours. She was experiencing discomfort in the region of her chest and shortness of breath that worsened markedly the more agitated she became.

I was working in the critical care area when she came in. Immediately, I thought to myself, *This woman doesn't look good.* I had a gut feeling that something was really wrong.

Her other doctors had attributed Julie's symptoms to a combination of anxiety and stress to her heart due to her obesity. The vagueness of her descriptions when she talked about her symptoms, combined with her age and the fact that she had been clinically diagnosed with anxiety several years before, made her current discomfort seem like a no-brainer for her doctors. She was having panic attacks, and her weight was compounding the issue. End of story.

However, as a specialist in sex and gender medicine, I knew that during myocardial infarction (MI)—aka, a heart attack—and other cardiovascular events, women often present much differently than men. In fact, women's cardiac symptoms are often described as "atypical" and "unusual" in medical literature. While men might experience pain radiating down the left arm, chest heaviness, or other stereotypical signs of a heart attack, women often present with only mild pain and discomfort, possibly combined with fatigue, shortness of breath, and a strong feeling that "something isn't right."

Julie was very pleasant, but I could tell she was scared. I calmly explained that, while her current issue *might* be exactly as other doctors had described, I would be more comfortable if we ordered an electrocardiogram (EKG) and blood work to make sure things looked normal.

When we got the results, I caught my breath. There was something very wrong here. *This could actually be a myocardial infarction,* I thought.

I immediately called our attending cardiologist. "I believe this woman is having an MI and needs to go to the cath lab," I told him. The cath lab is the medical suite where a procedure to fix blocked arteries is performed.

"A thirty-two-year-old woman?" There was a slight pause, then a sigh. "Oh, all right. I'll send someone down to take a look."

Like Julie's previous doctors, the cardiologist's assessment was that she was displaying symptoms of anxiety. But her EKG was slightly abnormal, so he finally agreed to take her to the cath lab.

About an hour later, I got a call from the cardiologist. "Dr. McGregor," the attending cardiologist began, sounding a bit astounded, "I wanted to let you know that your patient, Julie, had a 95-percent occlusion of her main coronary artery. We placed a stent to restore blood flow to her heart."

An occlusion of the main coronary artery, in a man, is often called a "widow maker." We see it all the time in men over fifty and in a number of postmenopausal women. And yet, here was sweet, thirty-two-year-old Julie presenting with a condition that was likely to kill her in weeks, if not days, if left untreated—and *no one had thought to look for it because her symptoms and risk factors weren't consistent with the classic male model of a heart attack.*

Thankfully, Julie pulled through the procedure and recovered. I didn't see her in the ED again, but her story has stayed with me. Sometimes, I wonder how many other women like her walk out the doors of other emergency departments every day without receiving the life-saving treatment they need and deserve. Even one is too many—but I have a feeling the number is much, much higher than that.

Our Modern Medical System Is Failing Women

The human mind built the automobile. It built televisions and computers and smartphones. When these things break, we understand how to fix them; we have an inventory of all the relevant components, diagrams of all the working parts.

But we didn't create our bodies. In some sense—whether you believe in evolution, natural selection, or intelligent design—our bodies are mystical. We are not developing them; we are merely trying to reveal how they work. And, in many ways, they are still beyond our ability to fully comprehend.

When we approach our bodies from a scientific perspective, we are therefore limited in our ability to hypothesize, study, test, and evolve our understanding. We have made massive strides in the last several decades, but in a sense, we still enter into every observation from a place of not having the full picture. We begin with a set of assumptions built on our prior research, but—as my work and that of others is beginning to prove—many of those assumptions may be erroneous.

One of the biggest and most flawed assumptions in medicine is this: if it makes sense in a male body, it must make sense in a female one.

In every aspect, our current worldwide medical model is based on, tailored to, and evaluated according to male models and standards. This is not an abstract statement or even an observation. It's a fact. All our methods for evaluating, diagnosing, and treating disease for both men and women are based on previous research performed on male cells, male animals, and male bodies. There are reasons our system has evolved this way, many of them scientifically reasonable. However, recent research is revealing that female bodies are physiologically different from men's on every level—from our chromosomes to our hormones to our bodily systems and structures. Therefore, the medicine that works for men doesn't always work for, or even apply to, women.

In the ED, I am on the front lines of medicine, and this gives me a unique perspective. I see a broad view of all aspects of health care and the conditions that many women live with every day. From infections to heart conditions, sprained ankles to strokes, head trauma to back pain, I see them all at play, in real time, across thousands of patients per year. More, I see how the current male-centric model of medicine is causing women to receive potentially inappropriate, ineffective, or even substandard care, every single day.

Women in cardiac distress don't receive the diagnostic tests they need because our protocols don't account for the way heart disease presents in women's bodies. Women are prescribed inappropriate doses of common medications because the initial drug trials didn't take into account the differences in female metabolism and hormonal cycles. All these issues, and more, contribute to poorer overall outcomes and higher mortality for women of all ages and backgrounds.

To me, Julie's case was significant because she actually presented with male-pattern heart disease, but in a distinctly female way. Women's symptoms are simply different from men's. They don't always have the classic male symptoms and pain profiles. Their symptoms often mimic other diseases and events that are considered more "female"—such as the panic attacks cited by Julie's previous doctors. Unfortunately, the difficulty she had in obtaining a diagnosis is all too common for women with cardiac issues, particularly younger women.

If a man comes into the ED with chest pain and shortness of breath, there's no question that he may be having an MI. If a woman comes in with the same issue, and she has a history of anxiety listed in her chart, the consensus will likely be that she's just suffering muscular and respiratory spasm related to anxiety. If her EKG comes back normal or close to normal, she'll be sent home. Although the symptoms she's exhibiting are strong potential indicators of female cardiac distress, our tests and protocols simply aren't designed to diagnose female patterns of disease, which tend to be more diffuse and uncharacterized than their male counterparts.

Discrepancies like these are what led me to specialize in sex and gender medicine in the first place. As a fresh-faced attending physician with a passion for women's issues and a strong calling to distinguish myself as a researcher in my chosen field, I found it fascinating that *researchers and specialists alike acknowledged both vast and subtle differences in symptomology, disease progression, and outcomes between men and women across the spectrum of physical and mental health—and yet no one was asking why such differences were present or how they might be affecting the way women were being cared for every day in both inpatient and outpatient settings and across all specialties.* Sex and gender differences in medicine weren't even being explored beyond the traditional scope of "women's health"—meaning, obstetrics and gynecology (OB/GYN) and breast health—let alone incorporated into the research and dialogue that ultimately shapes our medical procedures and policies in the ED and elsewhere.

Although I know that there are researchers like me working diligently to explore the difference in male and female physiology, the procedural and practical support necessary to put that knowledge into action isn't available to most emergency physicians when they show up to work. As a system, we simply aren't set up to give women the specialized care and treatment they need and deserve.

There are many reasons for this, which we will explore together in detail throughout this book. *The core issue, however, is that, despite decades of research and accumulated information, we are only just beginning to understand the scope of the differences between men and women and how those differences might impact everything from how drugs are prescribed, to how routine tests are performed, to how pain is assessed and treated, to how systemic disease is diagnosed.*

In other words, we need to reinvent modern medicine from the ground up to include the half of the human population it has, until now, marginalized and left behind.

The New Women's Health Revolution?

We are in the midst of a second women's revolution.

The first was the movement that gained women the right to operate in the world alongside men as legally equal human beings. We claimed the right to own and govern our bodies, our minds, and our property. We demanded the opportunity to pursue our educations, our passions, and our dreams. My mother's generation tore down the walls that, a mere fifty years ago, would have made my career in medicine and medical leadership challenging, if not impossible, to pursue.

The first revolution in women's health began in the 1970s with the publication of the groundbreaking book *Our Bodies, Ourselves*. This was the first time women were invited to understand themselves as biologically different from men. Women demanded access to things like birth control and pain relief. They realized that their bodies were not somehow flawed or "less than" simply because they were female. They demanded autonomy, and when the establishment resisted, they claimed it anyway.

Now, though, we need to call in another wave of change—a change based on the irrefutable facts available to us around women's health and women's bodies in all areas, not just in sexual and reproductive health.

Although we women have spent the last several decades fighting for equality, we are also becoming aware, sometimes painfully, that there *are* significant differences between men and women—differences for which our egalitarian vision did not account. These differences are at the heart of this new women's revolution, which is now coming to prominence.

Physiologically, neurologically, cognitively, socially, and experientially, women are unique. Every system in our bodies operates according to a biological imperative fine-tuned to our womanhood and the daily functions that womanhood necessitates. We are not simply men with breasts and ovaries—or, conversely, men who lack penises and testicles. We are not a genetic offshoot of men, as literal interpretations of scripture might imply. We are unique in every single cell of our bodies.

WHEN I FIRST STARTED my research on sex and gender differences in emergency medicine, I classified my work as "women's health." That made perfect sense to me, since I was literally researching the ways in which women's bodies operate and how their unique physiology influences diagnosis, disease progression, morbidity, pharmacological response, and other factors in health care. However, the outdated thinking around women's bodies is unbelievably pervasive; I wasn't prepared for how often others in my field would miscategorize and even misrepresent my work.

For most people—including the majority of medical professionals—"women's health" is synonymous with "reproductive health." OB/GYN and breast health immediately come to mind as areas of medical practice directly related to the health of women. (In fact, I spent much of my residency being called all over the ED to perform pelvic exams—not because no other doctor in the ED could do them, but because everyone thought that, as a women's health specialist, that would be my first priority. It still makes me laugh when I think about it!)

The truth is, women's health deals with exactly what the words, removed from their vernacular context, imply: *the overall health and well-being of women*. It is not simply about female reproductive organs, or pregnancy, or breast health, although those are all vital components. When I talk about women's health, I'm referring to the health of the *whole* woman, body and mind, with all the complexities inherent to a physiologically female body.

Every cell in a human body contains sex chromosomes. These chromosomes in turn influence every biological, chemical, sensory, and psychological function performed by that body. Most cells both produce and respond to sex hormones such as estrogen, progestins, testosterone, and androgens, and the functionality of each cell is affected in both subtle and overt ways by its relationship to these hormones.

Although these genomic differences have not been widely researched in all organs and systems, in areas where they have been studied, the implications are clear: women's bodies deal with everything from internal communication (neurotransmission) to external influences such as pharmaceuticals according to a different set of genetic and hormonal criteria. This means that what is considered medically "normal" for men may not be normal for—or even applicable to—women.

Here are a few common examples of how male-centric medicine impacts women's health every day:

- Coronary artery disease is the leading cause of death in both men and women, but women have statistically poorer outcomes and higher mortality in otherwise equivalent situations. A 2010 study found that "the under-recognition of heart disease and differences in clinical presentation in women lead to less aggressive treatment strategies and a lower representation of women in clinical trials."[1]
- Women are more likely to receive a psychiatric diagnosis for a multitude of conditions—including stroke, cardiac events,

irritable bowel syndrome, autoimmune disorders, and various neurological disorders—while men are more likely to be referred for tests.

- Men and women have markedly different responses and reactions to pain. Women have both a lower threshold for pain and a lower pain tolerance—meaning, they are more likely to perceive and report a lower level of discomfort as "pain" than men despite an equal degree of stimulation—however, the more vocal women become about their pain, the more likely their providers are to "tune them out" and prescribe either inadequate or inappropriate pain relief medication.
- Women often present with nontraditional symptoms of stroke, which causes delays in recognition by both them and their health professionals. When they get to the hospital, women experiencing stroke are less likely to receive rapid brain imaging. A European study found that, "Doppler examination, echocardiogram, and angiography were significantly less frequently performed in female than male patients.. They are also less likely to have echocardiography and carotid ultrasound performed during their stroke evaluation (important tools in both evaluating the cause of the stroke and preventing future episodes) or to receive treatment for acute stroke with the "clot-busting drug" called tPA (tissue plasminogen activator).[2]
- Women metabolize prescription drugs differently. For example, women experience greater adverse effects from using Ambien (zolpidem), a popular sleep aid, including morning sluggishness and impairment while driving. As it turns out, women only need half the originally recommended dose. Nearly twenty years after the drug's release, and after thousands of reports from patients who experienced adverse

effects, the Food and Drug Administration issued its first sex-specific prescribing guidelines.

And, of course, the current system routinely fails patients like Julie, whose doctors explained away her symptoms because, as a thirty-two-year-old woman, she didn't fit the "expected" pattern of cardiovascular disease they had learned in school. Across the country, every day, women like Julie come to their doctors with symptoms that don't fit a traditional male-centric pattern of disease. Sadly, many leave without answers—and, like Julie, might go days or weeks without the proper treatment for potentially deadly conditions.

My heart breaks when I consider how many women like Julie visit emergency departments across America every day and how few of them are statistically likely to get the treatment they need in a timely fashion—either because their symptoms don't fit a male paradigm or because their providers have an unconscious bias around women.

We need to wake up, individually and collectively, to the reality of being female in our current medical system. Only when we understand what's really going on can we make the fundamental changes necessary to improve women's outcomes. This isn't a single-layered issue of bias or faulty protocol. Every part of our current medical system—from research and analysis to medical education, from diagnostic testing to prescribing guidelines—needs to evolve at the same time, starting *now*.

This is a problem that can no longer be ignored. But while it may seem insurmountable, change *is* possible. By picking up this book, you have become part of the new women's health revolution. From now on, every time you speak to your doctor, every time you ask the right questions, every time you advocate for the right tests, you will be contributing to a landslide effect of awareness, improvement, and eventual reversal of our current male-centric paradigm. No effort is too small, no case too insignificant. Every time you advocate for the sex- and gender-specialized care that you and the women you love deserve, you will move our whole medical model one small step in the right direction.

Again, there's much more information to come, but for now I want you to understand this: *If you are a woman, you are at greater risk of misdiagnosis, improper treatment, and complications in common medical situations. To ensure that you receive the treatment you need and deserve, you need to understand how your body behaves differently from a man's and how to ask the simple questions that can mean the difference between a faulty or delayed diagnosis and lifesaving treatment.*

The medical world is evolving—however, like all revolutions, this one needs a "grassroots" component. I believe that the best way for women to effect immediate change in their health and health care is to advocate for themselves on both an individual and a collective basis, every day, starting now.

As I noted in the introduction, awareness and advocacy are the two keys to creating change from the ground up in our medical system: awareness because simply knowing that these issues exist for women in our healthcare system can help you get the treatment you need, and advocacy because, quite frankly, where attention goes in the medical world, research funding flows.

By picking up this book, you have become a standard-bearer. You will bring this new knowledge into your doctors' offices, hospitals, and urgent care centers and interact with your providers cooperatively, from a place of knowledge and empowerment. By advocating for your own health, asking for the tests, treatments, and prescriptions that will serve you best according to your individual health concerns, and referencing the details you will learn in this book and through your own research in conversations with your providers, you will directly impact your treatments, outcomes, and overall experiences, in the ED and elsewhere. By the time you turn the last page of this book, you will have all the information you need to approach this new conversation with your providers with confidence and clarity.

You Are Not a Statistic

In medicine, we often speak in broad terms, such as, "A team at the Technical University of Munich found that women are 1.5 times more likely to die in the first year after a heart attack than men."[3] This type of data helps researchers like me to see the big picture. But it doesn't speak to the human aspects of this higher mortality rate or the pain that these women and their families experience as a result.

I want to be clear that, although this book does look at broad-scope issues, *you are not a statistic*. You and the women you love matter. Your health matters. And your feelings matter.

I see the human cost of heart disease, stroke, pain disorders, neurological conditions, and trauma every day in my emergency department. I see the pain of families who have lost a mother, a sister, or a daughter to conditions that disproportionately affect women. I see women desperate for someone to listen to them, to believe them, because our male-centric medical model has classified their very real symptoms as "psychosomatic," "nonspecific," or "idiopathic" (meaning, of unknown origin).

I wrote this book not for our medical community but for you and the women you love. I want you to know and understand the differences in physiology that set women apart from men in ways that are more than just skin deep. And I want you to take this knowledge with you into your life and into your doctors' offices so that you too can be part of this medical revolution. Your contribution is crucial.

When you know how to ask the right questions, you can work with your providers to get the right care. Communication is a two-way street. We are no longer in the era of "doctor knows best." Yes, we physicians have dedicated a major chunk of our lives to understanding the human body and how it works—but in the end, no one knows your body better than you. With the tools in this book, you will become a partner in your own health care, and your provider will become not a dictator but an educated consultant who can help you decipher what's happening in your body and create a plan to address it. You can employ modern medicine in the way it was meant to be employed—as a tool for discovering, treating, and ultimately healing the physical and mental conditions that affect us as human beings.

What Matters—Your Key Takeaways

- Our male-centric medical model impacts women's health every day.
- If you are a woman, you are at greater risk of misdiagnosis, improper treatment, and complications in common medical situations. To ensure that you receive the treatment you need and deserve, you need to understand how your body behaves

differently from a man's and how to ask the simple questions that can mean the difference between a faulty or delayed diagnosis and lifesaving treatment. This book will show you how to do that.

- The most powerful tools for change in this arena are awareness and advocacy. Knowing how to ask the right questions can mean the difference between getting the treatment you need or being misdiagnosed, undertreated, or otherwise impacted by male-centric medicine.

chapter two

SEX IS MORE THAN SKIN DEEP

Not long after I applied for, and was granted, a research position at Brown University, I submitted a proposal for a didactic presentation at the annual meeting of the Society for Academic Emergency Medicine (SAEM). The presentation was titled "Women's Health and Gender-Specific Research in Emergency Medicine: Yesterday's Neglect, Tomorrow's Opportunities."

I was beyond excited about what I was discovering about women's bodies and their physiological and biochemical uniqueness, and I couldn't wait to share this with my peers. Surely, they would be as stunned and galvanized as I was.

Honestly, I was shocked that my proposal was accepted. I was a "newbie," a mere junior physician, barely out of my residency. Feeling empowered, I rounded up three experts to discuss sex and gender in relationship to emergency medicine. We all prepared our slides and notes and practiced our different roles in the presentation.

We flew out to Chicago for the meeting. I don't think I've ever been so nervous. This was my chance! I was going to start a conversation that would change emergency medicine forever!

Finally, it was time for our presentation. The previous didactic wrapped up, and the room was efficiently changed over. My colleagues and I came in with our notes and slides and set up quietly. The room was empty—but that was okay. People were coming from all over the hotel; it would take them time to arrive.

I fidgeted in my seat, watching the clock. Five minutes to go. Three. Two.

And then, it was time.

I looked out over a sea of empty chairs. The room was set up to hold sixty people, but only two seats were taken—one of them by my colleague and friend Dr. Libby Nestor and the other by my male officemate from Brown who'd stopped in to cheer me on before heading to the airport.

I had no idea what to do. My fellow presenters and I just sat there, staring at each other. Eventually, as if by unspoken consensus, we all stood and started packing our things. Our big idea, it seemed, was dead in the water.

This was such a powerful moment for me. Here was a conversation that could change the face of medicine as we knew it, something that could mean life or death for millions of women around the world—and *no one showed up*.

I understand now that my fellow physicians didn't skip my talk because they didn't care about women's health issues. They simply didn't know what they didn't know. In some respects, I was ahead of my time.

Research, education, and the work of actually providing care to patients are often treated as separate entities in our everyday medical reality. However, the knowledge that researchers gain is incorporated into medical education, which eventually has an effect on bedside care. If I wanted to create real, lasting change within modern medicine on behalf of women and their unique bodies, I would have to address all three of these areas simultaneously. I would have to educate researchers, inspire medical students, and serve my patients in a new, more enlightened way. My Sex and Gender Women's Health Collaborative has given me momentum to do exactly that, through fellowships, lectures, programs, meetings, and research.

In this chapter, I'll reveal the many ways in which the current medical establishment isn't set up to support women's bodies and how our flawed belief that women's bodies are equivalent to men's has negatively impacted women's outcomes at every level of care. We'll explore how, in every setting, from pharmaceutical laboratories to hospitals to physicians' offices, the male-centric model of medicine is ubiquitous and nearly unquestioned—and how understanding the impacts of this male "norm" can mean the difference between life and death for women around the world.

The Evolution of Male-Centric Medicine

Prior to the 1970s, medical research (and medical practice in general) was nowhere near as closely regulated as it is now. Today, every federally supported study and drug trial must be approved and monitored by an institutional review board to ensure that the study is ethical, presents minimal risks to participants, and is structured in accordance with solid scientific practices.

Fifty years ago, however, the world of medical research looked very different. It was essentially the Wild West of medicine. Every new drug was seen as likely to be beneficial and safe, and pharmaceuticals were tested and distributed with very little regulation. Clinical trials in the U.S. did not require approval by a review board; nor were they subject to oversight by any neutral party. In the U.K., the Medical Research Council was well-established, but its oversight had not evolved to the level we see today. The result was that Thalidomide's safety was vetted almost exclusively in animal trials before the drug was widely distributed to physicians.

This carefree approach changed drastically after numerous unforeseen consequences from new drugs and research impacted the health of tens of thousands of people. One example of this was the drug thalidomide. An anticonvulsive also marketed as a sleep aid and as a nausea reliever for pregnant women, thalidomide was available over the counter in Germany, and by prescription elsewhere. At first deemed safe and effective for all users, it was eventually determined to cause severe congenital malformations in fetuses—but not before vast numbers of pregnant women had innocently consumed it. Over 10,000 babies worldwide were born with missing or malformed limbs; damaged hearts, eyes, or digestive organs; and other major physical handicaps. Many survived only hours or days after birth. This tragedy, which affected families across Europe, Canada, and America, prompted an international investigation into drug research and human testing practices. The eventual outcome of this (and many other concurrent investigations) was the creation of the first "informed consent" laws for pharmaceutical trials in humans.

It wasn't until 1974 that protection for research subjects was written into law. In the U.S. the National Research Act created the National Commission for the Protection of Human Subjects of Biomedical and Behavioral Research, tasked with developing guidelines for medical research involving human subjects and regulating the use of human experimentation in medicine. Under this set of guidelines, pregnant women and women of childbearing age were considered "protected" subjects, and (unsurprisingly, given what had happened with thalidomide) many researchers opted to exclude them from their experiments altogether rather than jump through the hoops necessary to include them in a safe manner.

At the same time, as medical research evolved and became more regulated, researchers noticed that monthly female hormonal fluctuations created hard-to-account-for variables in their trials. Since expensive and time-consuming testing would be required to know where each woman was in her menstrual cycle at every point in the research timeline, many scientists opted to omit women altogether—both in human trials and in the initial phase of lab testing using animals.

Don't get me wrong: I am beyond grateful for the regulations and guidelines that keep women and babies safe from the potential complications of medical trials. *No one* should have to suffer in order to create a new drug or medical therapy—especially not mothers and their children. However, creating a "protected" status for premenopausal women has had the unforeseen effect of making the majority of medical research male centric. In an effort to protect women from the hazards of clinical trials, we have endangered them in another way.

The pervasive belief that women's bodies and systems are essentially the same as men's made this male-centric approach seem like a no-brainer in the beginning—but now that we know the difference, it's obvious that excluding half the population from clinical trials and drug-safety testing is not only a bad idea but a dangerous one.

Our current medical system favors male centrism at every level—from research planning, to funding and human trials, to implementation in hospital and outpatient settings. In order to show the scope of this issue, I've broken it down to demonstrate how all these various pieces come together to create a male-dominant, male-centric medical model.

- *Inception:* Every research study starts with an idea. For a research study to be approved, it needs to go through a series of institutional board reviews. Researchers need to prove that this study is not only valid from a medical point of view but can be conducted with minimal harm to people and animals. Because women of childbearing age were considered "protected" subjects under the National Research Act, and to some degree still are, this necessitates that female subjects undergo pregnancy testing, which on a large scale can be both expensive and time-consuming, and that female test subjects be educated on the risks of becoming pregnant during the study. Therefore, committees are more likely to approve research projects focused on male subjects or to suggest that a similar approach using male subjects be considered. In fact, a 2011 assessment of federally funded randomized clinical trials found that only 37 percent of participants were women. More, 64 percent of the studies examined "did not specify their results by sex and did not explain why the influence of sex in their findings was ignored."[1]

- *Funding:* All research needs funding. Funds can be obtained from a variety of sources, including institutions like hospitals, healthcare groups, and universities; government agencies; foundations like the American Heart Association or the

American Cancer Society; and industry or private donors. Because enrolling women in research trials necessitates extra costs, funding is more likely to be obtained for more "streamlined" male-model studies. Also, depending on their own donor demographic, some agencies are simply more likely to choose studies that benefit men.

- *Publication:* Once a research study is complete, it needs to be published in a medical journal to be disseminated. It needs to go through journal editors, then peer reviews to be published. This is a place where both explicit and implicit male bias can occur; consciously or not, journal editors tend to choose studies whose outcomes are important and interesting to them, and (at the time of this writing) most journal editors are male.

- *Education:* After the research is published, it will be used to educate doctors, nurses, and other medical professionals and inform patient-care decisions. However, the information in these studies is almost always presented as applicable to both men and women, regardless of what percentage (if any) of the study subjects were female, and regardless of whether sex was considered a "variable" in the research findings.

As you can see, from start to finish, our whole medical research process is based on a male paradigm. And time and time again, women have worse outcomes in areas of high public health significance.

The good news is, because there are so many steps in the research process, there are lots of places along the way to make change—but to create a landslide effect, we need to work in all of these areas simultaneously, as well as in the areas of drug research and development and medical education.

Our Current Medical Reality

Most of the time I don't get the information I need to treat patients successfully by looking at their medical charts. I get it by talking with them.

For example, if not for our conversation, I wouldn't have known that Rosita, who came in for chronic abdominal and pelvic pain, had been suffering her whole life with excruciatingly painful periods. When she'd consulted her general practitioner several years before, she had assumed the cause was "PMS," or premenstrual syndrome; her doctor had therefore suggested that she go home, take some ibuprofen, and rest with a heating pad. However, the pain increased with every period. Soon Rosita was missing whole days of work, driving to urgent care centers in search of pain relief, and praying for answers. But each time, the response was the same: "We aren't sure what's going on, so go home, rest, and follow up with your primary care doctor tomorrow." And each time, Rosita complied, though her intuition was screaming that something was wrong.

This particular month, she was bleeding even more heavily than usual and in so much pain she could barely walk. Desperate, she came into the emergency department. After our conversation, I sent her for an ultrasound.

As it turns out, Rosita's ultrasound had all the hallmarks of endometriosis. I recommended she follow up with a colleague of mine who specializes in that condition. Exploratory surgery confirmed the diagnosis; eventually, it was determined that Rosita needed a full hysterectomy.

I couldn't deduce this simply by looking at Rosita's chart because there was little relevant information to be found there. Our male-centric medical system doesn't address any of the subtleties of women's issues. We have blanket terms for women's symptoms (like PMS), but we don't have a system for delving into those issues in a way that can consistently result in accurate diagnoses. In fact, it takes an average of seven years in the U.S., and 7.5 years in the U.K., for a woman to obtain a diagnosis of endometriosis.[2]

While it may appear, from an outside perspective, that medicine is systemized to the last detail, this actually isn't true. Despite our incredible technologies and modern advances, much of diagnosis and treatment is still highly subjective—based on educated guesswork, theories, pattern recognition, and the occasional plain old-fashioned hunch—especially when it comes to women's health. In the ED, we often joke that "patients don't read the textbooks"—meaning that they rarely present in accordance with the classic teachings of how diseases manifest.

Doctors spend four years in medical school and three to six years in residency learning to put our vast body of knowledge into practice, and yet we still get caught off guard. We all have at least one story about someone who came into the ED with a sore throat and ended up needing surgery for appendicitis, or something else equally odd.

This indicates not that our textbooks have outlived their usefulness but rather that they are based upon historical averages that no longer fully apply. Most of the data used in medical education was compiled prior to the 1990s and reflects an era when patients waited to consult their doctors until something was "really wrong"—meaning, their disease had progressed significantly and had become more obvious with respect to diagnosis. Now, people tend to be more aware of their symptoms and to seek care for subtler issues; this is wonderful because it means that many potentially deadly diseases are caught in their early stages, but it also complicates diagnoses because, early in the disease process, the same symptoms can indicate multiple potential issues. For example, whereas people used to come into the ED with full-blown chicken pox (which was easy to diagnose), now they are coming in with a tiny red patch on the arm, which could be the first sign of chicken pox or anything from poison ivy to an allergic reaction. When we try to apply our textbook diagnostic training to unclear symptoms or early-stage disease, uncertainty ensues.

Things get even more convoluted when you factor in the many differences between men's and women's bodies. We can no longer ignore the evidence that a woman's every organ and system, from her brain to her bones, from her metabolism to her arteries and veins, is physiologically unique—and that, as such, she must be offered different and appropriate diagnoses, treatments, and preventive care. However, I and my contemporaries didn't even *have* textbooks for this kind of thing in med school. At least, not until the textbook, *Sex and Gender in Acute Care Medicine*, for which I was the lead editor, was published. Everything we learned in school was based on the male-centric model, and every procedure we learned was based on male-centric care. Most anatomy books used in medical schools around the world only male models, providing disembodied breasts and pelvises when female "parts" are discussed. Mannequins used for simulations in academic settings are male; usually, the only available female model is a pregnant one. Even our electronic medical records use photos of male models. In the ED, we literally have to use pictures of men while we attempt to illustrate female patterns of pain and disease to women!

Different groups of women are also at higher risk in our healthcare system because of lack of research. For example, many drug trials and research studies do not include elderly patients because such patients tend to take too many other prescriptions, which can confound study results, or because diseases like dementia and stroke prevent the patient from giving informed consent. However, since this is the population that will most likely be using the drugs and protocols being researched in these trials, we are left with a huge margin of error.

Women of color are also overlooked in research despite their unique risk factors and so continue to suffer unacceptable outcomes across the board.[3] We'll talk about this unacceptable disparity in greater detail in Chapter 8, but for the purposes of this discussion, it's vital to note that, in 2017, the Center for Drug Evaluation and Research approved over forty-five new drugs, which had been studied in over 60,000 participants. Only 7 percent of those participants (of both genders) were black or African American, and only 14 percent were Hispanic. A 2016 article in *The Atlantic* noted, "Since 1993, fewer than 5 percent of respiratory studies funded by the National Institute of Health have included reports on racial or ethnic minorities… and fewer than 2 percent funded by the National Cancer Institute have met diversity goals."[4]

And, as noted, pregnant women are ignored by research trials completely; in fact, they are often referred to as "therapeutic orphans." Of course, no one wants to create another horrible situation like what we saw with thalidomide—and, thankfully, our current knowledge and protocols would never allow that to happen. But neither is it acceptable only a handful of medications are widely considered "safe" for use during pregnancy, most of them related to the pregnancy itself, all of them for conditions related to the pregnancy itself (nausea, labor complications, and pain). Pregnant women get sick, and sick women get pregnant—but because of our reluctance to study pregnant women, the drugs they take for their conditions come with an unknown set of risks. Women are then left to choose between treating their own serious or even life-threatening condition and protecting their infant's health. This not only is unacceptable in human terms but also puts women at risk for the very same unforeseen complications we have been trying to avoid. Even Tylenol, which is considered the only "safe" pain reliever to use during pregnancy and nursing, has not been evaluated in controlled studies with pregnant women. The only difference is that, because most medications have not been studied, the risks (and blame) for adverse effects fall on the women themselves, who often have no idea that the medicines they are taking for their asthma, hypertension, depression, anxiety, or seizures could pose a risk to their babies.

The fact is that, despite all the scientific advances we've made in the last forty years, women still experience poorer outcomes in all areas of health, and women of color experience worse outcomes than white women. Women in general are less likely than men to be treated for lots of things—for sepsis, for myocardial infarction, for stroke, for arrhythmia. Women also struggle to receive appropriate diagnoses and treatment for women-specific diseases like endometriosis and for chronic pain conditions like fibromyalgia. And women are less likely to be treated appropriately for that great equalizer: pain.

THE LACK OF WIDELY AVAILABLE INFORMATION and education is frustrating for physicians who just want to help their patients. I've actually coined the term "undiagnosed women's disease," or "UWD," to cover the multitude of cases that our current tools can't help us diagnose and treat. In her book *Doing Harm*, Maya Dusenbery called this lack of understanding of women's medical conditions "medically unexplained symptoms." The Office of Research on Women's Health at the National Institutes of Health refers to women as "the three U's": understudied, underdiagnosed, and undertreated.

If you've noticed a theme here, you're right. Across every area of health care, women are less researched, less understood, and quite literally less cared for than men.

One problem is that many providers aren't comfortable with a diagnosis as vague as "UWD." They want to give a name to what's wrong, and their patients want answers. So they default to the diagnosis that makes the most sense at the moment, even if it's not actually a good fit, just to have some parameters to put around the situation. Such diagnoses are often of "syndromes," which is a wastebasket term for a collection of symptoms without an underlying etiology (known cause).

Rosita's diagnosis of premenstrual syndrome is a perfect example of this. PMS is a collection of symptoms attributed to the event of monthly menstruation but without a known underlying causation. This was the closest her providers could come to what was happening to her without a battery of invasive tests, so that was the diagnosis she was given.

In order to receive an accurate diagnosis and lifesaving treatment, a woman will often need to convince her provider—despite previous diagnoses to the contrary—that something is actually wrong. Women with microvascular disease may have perfectly normal stress tests but suffer from terrible recurring chest pain; those same women could drop dead of a heart attack a week later with nothing on their medical charts to indicate that they were at risk. Woman having strokes can present with headaches and dizziness without the standard (read: male-pattern) droopy face and weak extremities;

because providers don't know how to recognize female-pattern symptoms, women having strokes often fail to receive critical interventions like tPA (the powerful clot-busting drug).[5] Women with lung and ovarian cancers (two of the top cancer killers of women, both more likely to be lethal than breast cancer) may present with few, if any, definitive symptoms until it's too late and the cancer has metastasized.[6] And all along the way, doctors without access to critical gender-based information are treating them for the wrong things, unable to diagnose them at all—or, worse, brushing off their symptoms as "all in their heads."

This points not only to our inability to properly diagnose women physically but also to the gender and cultural biases women face in our medical system—from both male and female doctors. The perception of how women experience pain and the management of women's pain both in and out of a hospital setting are highly problematic. Women of color are even more likely to have their pain minimized; one study found that "African Americans and Hispanics were less likely than white patients to receive any pain medication and more likely to receive lower doses of pain medication, despite higher pain scores."[7]

Women are also more likely to receive a psychiatric diagnosis when they report their symptoms, regardless of the nature of those symptoms. As several writers have observed, the words "hysteria" and "hysterical" are derivatives of the Greek word for uterus, *hystera*. While formal diagnoses of hysteria are thankfully a thing of the past, there is still a pervasive unconscious belief in the medical culture that women are prone to illogical and unreasonable outbursts. Then, when women express their pain and distress, their complaints are taken less seriously because they are perceived as less likely to be a product of physical disease.

Given the knowledge we currently have about the differences between men and women, one might think that there would exist at least a general set of protocols and criteria for medical professionals to apply when diagnosing and treating women. Unfortunately, this is not the case. Most drug trials, testing, and research studies have been (and in many cases continue to be) performed exclusively on men. Our testing and treatment protocols are developed to identify male-pattern symptoms. The foundational research on which our new experiments are based is still male centric and male dominated. And despite the growing body of evidence to the contrary, the majority of the medical world continues to assume that, with the exception of their sex organs, men and women are biologically identical.

The combination of cultural and procedural bias with the reliance on a male model for scientific inquiry has rendered our current medical system male centric. And while few practitioners consciously subscribe to the illogic and scientific inequality that has contributed to the creation of that system, they are nevertheless operating within it and according to its rules. The result is that women whose conditions or experiences don't line up with male models are at increased risk of receiving inappropriate, inferior, or even injurious care.

It's a huge problem—one I'm working diligently every day to solve.

In my tenure as an emergency medicine specialist, educator, and researcher, I have observed six key areas where the biological, biochemical, and biopsychological variations between men and women have created blatant and potentially harmful misalignments in diagnosis, testing, and treatment both inside and outside the emergency department. These areas are as follows:

- Cardiac and stroke diagnosis and treatment in women
- Prescription and dosing of pharmaceuticals
- Subjective evaluation of women's symptoms (including the role of mental health diagnoses)
- Pain and pain management
- Hormones and female biochemistry (including prescribed hormones)
- Gender, cultural, and societal conventions, including LGBTQ/ transgender issues

In Part II of this book, you will learn more about each of these six major areas of health where women consistently deal with misdiagnoses, inadequate treatment, and poorer outcomes. Each chapter will include not only powerful stories and discussion of specific diseases and treatments but also critical information about potential symptoms, warning signs, and women-specific treatment options that will empower you to have better conversations with your providers and increase your likelihood of receiving appropriate, potentially lifesaving care.

By the time you turn the last page of this book, you will have all the information you need to approach this new conversation with your providers with confidence and clarity.

Every day brings progress. But until the medical establishment catches up with the science, *it's up to you to take a more active role in advocating for yourself and your loved ones. Only in this way can you have immediate influence on your care and see immediate results.*

In other words, it's time to join our Women's Health Revolution.

What Matters—Your Key Takeaways

- Every area of our medical world has evolved to be male centric in a multitude of ways.
- Women are underserved, understudied, underdiagnosed, and undertreated in multiple areas of high public health significance—including cardiac disease, stroke, cancer, and pain disorders, as well as women-specific conditions. If you are a woman, you are at greater risk of misdiagnosis, improper treatment, and complications in common medical situations.
- Women are underrepresented in clinical and pharmaceutical research trials, and most trials do not account for sex differences as a variable.
- Some populations of women—like pregnant mothers, the elderly, and women of color—are even less represented than women in general and have measurably poorer outcomes.
- Doctors often don't have the tools necessary to diagnose female expressions of common health conditions.

PART TWO

THE SIX BIGGEST ISSUES FACING WOMEN'S HEALTH TODAY

chapter three

WOMEN'S HEARTS (AND BRAINS) BREAK DIFFERENTLY

Some of the most dramatic moments in the emergency department happen when cardiac patients come in.

Often, it's just what you would expect to see on a TV show: a middle-aged or older man lying limp on a stretcher, an emergency medical technician (EMT) astride him doing chest compressions while the nurses wheel him through the doors. But for women, the situation often looks far different.

One day a few years ago, a woman came in on a stretcher in the late evening. She was pale, sweating, and gasping for breath—all signs of flash pulmonary edema or sudden heart failure. She was younger than I would have expected for someone with these symptoms—in her mid-fifties—and while slightly overweight, not obese. The friend who'd followed the ambulance to the ED told the intake staff that my patient had suddenly collapsed over dinner in one of Providence's trendy restaurants.

Once the patient, whose name was Sharin, was admitted and stabilized, she was sent to the cath lab for testing. I had a moment to speak with her friend, who was huddled in her chair in the waiting area.

"I don't know what happened," the friend sobbed. "One minute, she was fine. The next, she was keeling over!"

"Did Sharin have any heart troubles before this?" I asked. There was nothing on her chart except an anxiety diagnosis, but given how commonly women's heart disease is misdiagnosed, I always like to get the other side of the story.

"Not that I know of," the friend replied. "She's healthy! She works out every day."

"How about stressful events in her life recently?"

"Well, her husband died a few weeks ago. It was unexpected. She's got two kids in college and one still at home. She's kind of in shock." The friend dissolved into tears again. "I was just taking her out to dinner to cheer her up!"

My heart went out to her—and to Sharin, who was suddenly facing a future full of uncertainty.

After asking an aide to help settle the friend, I called our cath lab. "Have you done the angiogram yet?" I asked. "I think we may have a case of Takotsubo's here."

Takotsubo cardiomyopathy, also known as "stress cardiomyopathy" or "broken heart syndrome," primarily affects women. After a stressful or traumatic event, the body experiences a massive rise of catecholamines (aka, the "fight or flight" hormones). All of a sudden, the left ventricle of the heart is stunned and balloons outward, and the heart can no longer beat very well. Often, the patient will experience intense, angina-like pain in the chest area; other times, she will collapse completely.

The name Takotsubo comes from the Japanese *tako–tsubo*, which means "fishing pot for trapping octopus"; when this condition is present, the swelling of the left ventricles causes the heart to take on that distinctive fishing-pot shape.

In Sharin's case, the shock and stress of losing her husband had caused her stress hormones to skyrocket. Thankfully, Takotsubo's is transient and, with proper supportive care and medication, will often resolve in a few days or weeks. However, if the underlying cause of the stress is not addressed, women who experience Takotsubo's are at risk for other incidences of cardiac failure in the future.

Sharin didn't come back to the ED but was instead sent up to a room in the main hospital for supportive care and observation. I hoped that she would not only recover from her sudden heart failure but also receive what she needed to process what had happened and grieve for her husband. I hoped she would heal and be there for her kids.

This is the hard part, for me, of working in the ED. My job is to tackle the acute issues of the moment and then send my patients to the specialists who can care for them in the longer term. I get the story of the illness but not always the full story of the healing.

Sharin's case stuck with me in large part because of her anxiety diagnosis. There is a huge overlap between heart disease and anxiety diagnoses in women. Takotsubo cardiomyopathy, in particular, seems to strike women with anxiety more heavily. One small study found that "in comparison to background controls, TTC [Takotsubo] patients reported significantly less well-being, more neuroticism, more depression, and more anxiety."[1]

41

This made sense to me. Of course women with previous anxiety would be more prone to a condition triggered by extreme levels of stress hormones. But what about other heart conditions? Was anxiety an underlying cause—or just the default diagnosis for a pattern of chronic and subtle female heart disease that our male-centric model doesn't understand?

Do We Really Understand Women's Heart Disease?

Women are far less likely than men to fit the textbook model of heart disease—but they are also more likely to die of a cardiac event. In fact, according to a study published in the *Journal of the American Heart Association*, they are up to *three times more likely* to die after a serious heart attack than men.[2] That is a staggering statistic—especially when you consider that the common perception is still that heart attacks are a "men's disease."

What's more, the Centers for Disease Control and Prevention reports that 64 percent of women who die suddenly of a heart attack (or heart attack–like event) exhibited no previous symptoms.[3] I don't disagree with the statistic, but "exhibited no previous symptoms" doesn't mean there were no red flags. It simply means that no symptoms that fit with the male model of heart disease were reported.

In general, we know that women are less likely to have "traditional" heart attacks—meaning, the myocardial infarctions, or "widow makers," that create the classic symptoms of acute chest and left arm pain. In fact, women are more likely to describe "chest discomfort" when having a heart attack; this may be a diffuse ache, pressure, or "just a funny feeling" rather than the stereotypical

42

"elephant on my chest." They are also more likely than men to present with a cluster of symptoms such as shortness of breath, unusual fatigue (sometimes for days or weeks before the actual cardiac event), nausea, digestive issues, or even "brain fog." Alone or in combination, none of these things scream "heart attack" to women because they, too, are expecting themselves to exhibit the standard male patterns of heart disease!

Often, when women finally do call 911 or drive themselves to the ED, they don't receive the proper interventions. There is often a delay between ambulance pickup and arrival at the hospital, perhaps because the EMTs don't recognize the symptoms or urgency, or perhaps because the women themselves downplay what's happening—we don't know for sure. When women get to the hospital, there's a delay in first medical contact, because they aren't seen as priority cases. Diagnostic tests like angiograms, angioplasty, cardiac catheterization, and stress tests/electrocardiograms (EKGs)—all of which are designed to look for male-pattern disease—often come back with negative or inconclusive results. They may be told that the tightness in their chest is musculoskeletal or that they are just having a really strong panic attack and should go home and relax because nothing is wrong with their hearts. Regardless of what causes the delay, however, the longer the time lapse between the first sign of a heart attack and the application of appropriate interventions, the less likely a woman is to have a positive outcome.

In order to help women get the treatment they need and deserve, we need to learn to recognize the symptoms of female-pattern disease.

The first thing we need to understand is that women's hearts don't "break" the same way as men's. Instead of presenting with the textbook-pattern blocked big blood vessels, which can be resolved through the implantation of stents or through surgery, women's heart disease tends to be more diffuse. While men have plaque that builds up in their blood vessels and eventually ruptures (causing myocardial infarction or similar events), women's plaque erodes *into* the blood vessels, making them stiffer and less flexible. When dye is injected during an angiogram, we may not see the typical types of clot formations in women because the plaque is in the lining of the vessels themselves. Then, when no areas of clotting show up in the images, the threat of vascular disease is minimized or ruled out entirely, when in fact it's simply manifesting in a different, woman-specific way. Women then experience yet another level of misdiagnosis and delay in treatment.

Coronary microvascular dysfunction—also referred to as "microvascular disease" or "small vessel disease"—is a condition in which the small blood vessels around the heart become damaged or weakened; this restricts blood flow to and from the heart, resulting in spasms of and stress to the heart muscle. Microvascular disease is far more common among women than men, potentially because our blood vessels tend to be smaller and therefore more susceptible to damage. This condition is also extremely hard to diagnose because our standard tests (angiogram and EKG) aren't designed to detect it. Nor has there been extensive research about how to treat it; the only pharmaceuticals available are the typical antihypertensives and cholesterol-lowering drugs, so we are forced to treat the condition with what we have available and simply wait to see what happens.

The result of this lack of knowledge is that many women with this dangerous condition never even learn that they have it until they have a full-blown heart attack—and, as we've seen in this discussion, sometimes not even then. Sharonne Hayes, MD, professor of cardiovascular medicine at the Mayo Clinic, observed in an interview with Randy Young that "some women with microvascular disease who complain of angina feel they must be crazy and should see a psychiatrist because their doctor says there is nothing wrong with them. It reaches a point where they're not just undertreated but under-believed."[4]

There is hope on this front, however. C. Noel Bairey Merz, MD, director of the Barbra Streisand Women's Heart Center, is leading the charge to change women's heart health care and research. Her research is focused on creating in-clinic solutions for patients who have chest pain but no visible arterial blockage, examining the relationship between estrogen levels and heart disease, and encouraging more women to participate in clinical trials. Her clinical trials have already revealed that a magnetic resonance imaging (MRI) stress test is superior to standard angiogram or EKG testing to reveal coronary microvascular dysfunction; we hope that this will soon be integrated into protocol nationwide as a lifesaving strategy for diagnosing women's heart disease.

Basmah Safdar, MD, is an emergency medicine physician who is also working to serve the women who come into her ED repeatedly for chest pain but exhibit normal stress tests and angiograms. She is researching the physiology of coronary microvascular dysfunction using cardiac positron emission tomography, which can show important metabolic changes in an organ or blood vessel right down to the cellular level. Examining the relationship between patients who have recurrent chest pain and coronary microvascular dysfunction can reveal other vascular-related conditions that are more common in women, such as kidney failure, obesity, sleep disorders, dementia, and diabetes. Dr. Safdar hopes to make it possible for women to get the treatment they need before they have a life-threatening cardiac event. Dr. Safdar told me,

> Having talked to many women with long-standing chest pains, I now believe that identifying small vessel disease of the heart is critical. It not only validates the symptoms of patients who have been suffering for a long time and helps us start correct treatment in these patients by making the right diagnosis, but importantly it allows us to recognize patients at risk for failure of multiple organ systems, as small vessel disease is often not limited to the heart only. It is only a matter of time before other organs such as the brain or the kidneys start showing signs of the disease as well. We must take steps to recognize early and take steps to slow the progression of this debilitating disease.

Women Have Unique Risk Factors for Heart Disease

Women don't just exhibit different symptoms and manifestations of heart disease than men, they also have different risk factors.

While traditional risk factors—like hypertension, high cholesterol, diabetes, obesity, and smoking—are still relevant to women, the physiological differences in women still require extensive study. For example, we know that conventional risk factors have different "weights" for men and women: while smoking is a statistically greater risk factor for cardiac disease in women than in men, hypertension is a greater risk factor for men than women. What we don't know is how factors like hormone levels, fat distribution, and metabolism affect and predict women's heart disease.

There are also risk factors unique to women that are only now being introduced into the general body of literature. Researchers recently uncovered a link between heart disease and perinatal and peripartum complications like preeclampsia, eclampsia, intrauterine growth retardation, and gestational diabetes; women who experience these issues during pregnancy often have greater levels of systemic inflammation, which puts them at greater risk for coronary disease.[5]

Autoimmune diseases like rheumatoid arthritis are also being looked at as correlating factors for heart disease in women because of the link between inflammation and microvascular disease. In a 2017 article, the Cleveland HeartLab observed, "The process doesn't stop at the joints. The inflammation can damage systems throughout the body, including the skin, eyes, lungs, and heart. Inflammation narrows the arteries, raising blood pressure and reducing blood flow to the heart, for instance. No wonder people with rheumatoid arthritis have a 50 percent higher risk of experiencing a heart attack, twice the rate of heart failure, and more peripheral vascular disease than those without the condition."[6] A review of studies published in the journal *Nature Reviews Rheumatology* offered another startling statistic: findings suggested that more than 50 percent of premature deaths in patients with rheumatoid arthritis resulted from cardiovascular conditions. As it happens, 75 to 78 percent of those with rheumatoid arthritis are women.[7]

At the time of this writing, the American Heart Association has updated its clinical practice guidelines to include some of this information. However, the differing risk factors and risk factor weights and the common presentation of symptoms for women have not been included. In fact, beyond the piece about pregnancy complications, very little about sex and gender differences has been addressed at all. This is highly problematic.

Without the proper tests to identify women-specific heart issues like microvascular dysfunction, doctors are left to tell their patients, "Your angiogram and cardiac catheterization are normal, so...maybe it's your anxiety."

In other words, women are once again hearing, "It's all in your head."

Anxiety Complicates Women's Heart Diagnoses

There is also the issue of anxiety, which is the second-most-diagnosed mental disorder in American women.[8] Severe panic attacks and actual cardiac events look very similar at first glance. I often wonder how many of those women with anxiety diagnoses who experienced fatal heart attacks actually had coronary microvascular dysfunction or some other female variant of heart disease but were never diagnosed. It's impossible to know for sure at this juncture; such data has not been collected.

What *is* clear is that people with an anxiety diagnosis are statistically more likely to have a heart attack—and women are more than twice as likely as men to have an anxiety disorder.[9] In fact, one study from Tilburg University in Holland looking at the combined data of over 250,000 people found that those who experienced frequent anxiety were 26 percent more likely to have coronary disease and 48 percent more likely to die from heart-related issues. Another study conducted in Sweden concluded that anxiety more than doubled the risk of heart attack in subjects.[10]

The question then becomes, *Do women have heart disease because they have anxiety—or do they have heart disease that is causing anxiety-like symptoms and being misdiagnosed?*

As our understanding of women's heart disease evolves, I hope that we will find definitive answers to these questions and create new protocols and evaluation tools to help women treat their unique expressions of heart disease earlier and more effectively. Unfortunately, tests that specifically look for microvascular disease are evolving and are not readily available—but thanks to the work of my colleagues Dr. C. Noel Bairey Merz and Dr. Basmah Safdar, they will hopefully be commonplace in all EDs within a few years.

In the meantime, however, my recommendation is that all women with anxiety who experience or have experienced heart attack–like symptoms (panic attacks, shortness of breath, chest pain, etc.) request a thorough evaluation of their cardiac health, including the following:

- EKG
- Inflammatory marker blood tests
- Full assessment and reduction of traditional and nontraditional risk factors
- A stress test if the risk factor assessment determines that the symptoms are cardiac in origin (Ask for a stress test directly if you feel that your symptoms are heart related.)

These will help you and your doctor begin to discern whether anxiety is causing your symptoms or heart disease is causing your anxiety.

Finally, it's important to remember that all protocols in the medical world have some element of gestalt—meaning that the practitioner is expected to apply his or her own judgment to the situation, organizing all the various pieces of information into a theory that represents the whole picture for the patient. Even in the most rigorous protocol for treating someone in cardiac distress, there's room for the physician to question whether the way the patient is presenting is congruent with a heart attack. The fact that there's room for professional judgment is a good thing—but the flip side is that there is also room for unconscious bias.

Anxiety, in this sense, is a tripwire for gestalt. Anxiety is stigmatized in our society, and people who have it are often portrayed as inherently weaker or less objective than those who don't. When a physician doesn't have an explanation for a woman's symptoms and doesn't have all the information about how women's heart disease manifests differently than men's, anxiety is often the easy diagnosis—even when it's not the whole story.

We'll explore the topic of anxiety overdiagnosis further in Chapter 5, but for now, my advice is to trust yourself and not minimize your symptoms or second-guess what you're feeling.

I have a talk that I give to all my female students. I call it the "Stop Apologizing Talk." Women say "I'm sorry" for everything, even when they have nothing to be sorry for. If you struggle with anxiety and are exhibiting any of the symptoms of heart disease we've discussed, stop apologizing for your symptoms and seek the care you need.

The first step is to have a candid talk with your provider. You might say something like, "I feel like this is different from my normal anxiety. Is there another possible explanation for these symptoms?" or "I've had panic attacks before, and this is different. Can we talk about whether a stress test is appropriate for me?" These types of question can open up a conversation around what your provider is thinking and why he or she has come to certain conclusions about your symptoms.

Be honest, clear, and as detailed as possible. Remember, your doctor doesn't necessarily have all the information about your health history (especially if you see multiple providers). You might consider putting together a "CliffsNotes" (or, for the Millennial generation, "SparkNotes") version of your health history, including your medications, past health history, surgical history, and even any vitamins or herbal supplements you're taking. Then ask your doctor to compare it to what's in your chart and explain why you think you're experiencing something more than just run-of-the-mill anxiety or stress-related symptoms.

If you feel like you need some support or aren't sure which questions to ask, consider bringing a friend or relative with you. They can be more objective and may ask questions you hadn't thought of.

The best thing you can do for your heart is to start the conversation.

Women's Heart Disease Is Not Treated Like Men's

We now understand how women's heart disease manifests differently than men's and why it can be more difficult for our current tests and protocols to diagnose. But what about the women who already know that they have heart disease? Are they the lucky ones experiencing better outcomes?

Sadly, the answer is no. Our male-centric model is failing them as well.

Remember Julie from Chapter 1? I wish that I could say that her close call due to repeated misdiagnosis of her arterial occlusion was unusual, but it wasn't. Cases like hers happen every day in emergency departments and doctors' offices across America. Julie's case is so interesting because the presentation of her symptoms was, in fact, "typical" of the male-centric model. It's just that no one expected to see the typical symptoms of a sixty-five-year-old male manifesting in a thirty-two-year-old woman's body.

According to the World Heart Federation, women are less likely to receive the same diagnostic tests as men *even when they exhibit the same or similar symptoms*; as a result, their heart disease is 50 percent more likely to be misdiagnosed initially.[11] (Often, this will result in an anxiety diagnosis!) And despite procedural and prescription guidelines that suggest such treatments are valid for both genders, women are 34 percent less likely to undergo procedures like bypass surgery, stent implantation, and other procedures to clear arterial blockages; 16 percent less likely to receive a recommendation for aspirin therapy; and 24 percent less likely to receive a prescription for a statin (cholesterol-lowering) drug. The same study found that when this treatment gap was closed, women's mortality results improved dramatically, to the point where they were nearly equivalent to men's.

Another study, which looked at men and women with a form of heart failure referred to as heart failure with reduced ejection fraction (HFrEF), concluded rather bluntly that "although women with HFrEF live longer than men, their additional years of life are of poorer quality, with greater self-reported psychological and physical disability. The explanation for this different sex-related experience of HFrEF is unknown as is whether physicians recognize it. Women continue to receive suboptimal treatment, compared with men, with no obvious explanation for this shortfall."[12]

In short, women are not getting the same treatment or quality of care as men. And despite the fact that this disparity in outcomes is widely recognized and documented, no one seems to know *why* it keeps happening.

Part of the issue is that researchers are not educated enough about sex differences to consider crucial variables in risk factors and female patterns of disease. It's simply assumed that a heart is a heart and that the results and statistics that apply to men will naturally apply to women as well.

I saw a perfect example of this misconception on a CBS morning show in 2015. A well-known physician commentator was discussing a study that showed that good cardiac health (as determined by EKG/stress tests) in middle-aged men predicted not only a lower rate of cardiac death over the next ten years but also a lower rate of lung and colorectal cancer. When asked if the study included women, he replied, "This study just happened to look at men. One would assume that the results would be similar in women [but] that study hasn't been announced or looked at yet."[13] Even this renowned doctor was apparently unaware that women at severe risk for cardiac events can still present with "normal" stress test results.

That the results of all-male studies are being applied to women so offhandedly should be alarming—but within the medical community, this sort of thing happens all the time. Moreover, inviting the public to assume that stress tests are a major indicator of future good health is not only incorrect but dangerous.

If you're tempted to say, "But that was years ago!" trust me, this type of thing is still happening. I recently read a study published in the *Journal of the American Medical Association (JAMA) Cardiology* detailing the results of a fifteen-year study on the relationship between heart disease and exercise.[14] This study was also referenced in a *New York Times* article, which noted, "The researchers focused on the records of 21,758 men, most of them in their 50s. (They did not include women but plan to in a follow-up study.)"[15]

I could only shake my head and ask myself, *Why are women always an afterthought?*

Misperceptions about women and how they experience heart disease also contribute to how, when, and to what degree women's cardiac issues are treated. A great example of this is the way chest pain units are run in hospitals.

A chest pain unit—or its U.K. equivalent, the Rapid Access Chest Pain Clinic—is pretty much what it sounds like. It's a section of the hospital where people who are having chest pain (or other traditional symptoms associated with cardiac events) are sent for observation and testing. If you come into the hospital with symptoms that might be a heart attack, but it's not clear to the ED physicians that you are actually *having* a heart attack, you will be sent to the chest pain unit for twenty-four hours or so. You'll get repeated bloodwork and EKGs and maybe a stress test. If it's apparent that something is going on, you'll be sent to the cardiac ward. If not, you'll be sent home.

The purpose of the chest pain unit is, ostensibly, to provide a safety net to patients who may be having a major cardiac event but aren't necessarily in imminent danger or showing the classic symptoms. However, when you look at who is eligible to go to the chest pain unit, it's easy to see that this entire system and all its attendant protocols are built according to a male-centric model.

While both men and women can exhibit chest pain during a heart attack, there's also a group of people who don't have chest pain. This group does include men but, statistically, comprises predominantly women. Both men and women who have a heart attack without that key symptom of chest pain tend to have worse outcomes across the board because they almost always experience a delay in recognition and treatment.

When it comes to who gets sent to the chest pain unit for testing and observation, several criteria inform an ED doctor's decision. Blood enzyme levels, EKG results, and other factors (many of which we know are not always accurate indicators of heart attack in women) are considered. There's also a gestalt factor, which basically asks the doctor, "How likely do you think it is that this person's symptoms are from heart disease?" This subjective assessment is where many mistakes and oversights happen. Doctors are only human, after all.

The difference between male- and female-pattern heart attacks means that women are less likely to be admitted to the chest pain unit and more likely to be sent home without additional intervention. The protocols for observation and testing simply aren't set up to look for female-pattern symptoms—and so, even women whose hearts are in imminent danger might be sent home with no diagnosis and inconclusive test results.

Even when women are admitted to the chest pain unit, they are less likely to receive the same tests as their male counterparts.

I conducted a study of chest pain unit admissions along with my colleagues Esther K. Choo, MD, and Anthony M. Napoli, MD. We found that "a physicians' gender may impact test utilization in the diagnosis of acute cardiovascular disease."[16] For example, male physicians appeared less likely to use stress testing in female patients even after controlling for clinical variables. This indicates a disparity in decision making that is correlated with the interaction between male physicians and female patients.

Since cardiologists are the last stop on the decision train for patients in the chest pain unit, they are ultimately the ones who decide whether a patient stays for additional testing or gets sent home. And because a substantial piece of this assessment is subjective, there is room for inherent bias—or a simple lack of understanding about how female-pattern cardiac disease presents—to create a situation where a woman's heart attack or cardiac dysfunction is overlooked, misdiagnosed, or undertreated.[17]

The final factor that creates poorer outcomes for women with heart disease is the treatment they receive post–heart attack. In her article "The Way to Women's Heart Health," Randy Young writes,

"According to an AHA scientific statement on acute myocardial infarction (AMI) in women, 'although referral to CR [cardiac rehabilitation] is designated as a performance measure of healthcare quality after AMI, CR has failed to reach more than 80 percent of eligible women in the last three decades.'"[18] When women do receive rehabilitative treatment, it appears to be less comprehensive than that offered to men.

Women's Heart Disease Is Not Studied Like Men's

Despite the fact that heart disease is the number one killer of women, women are still not being included in proportionate numbers in large heart disease trials. In fact, on average, only about 30 percent of cardiac trial participants are women. And even when women take part in larger numbers, very few of those studies are designed to conduct sex-specific analysis—so the fact that we are enrolling more women doesn't mean we are getting more or better information. In fact, the information we're getting is *reinforcing* the male-centric model of heart disease diagnosis and treatment, not reversing it.

Here's a great example of this. When a man having a cardiac arrest comes into the ED, it's often a scene like what I described at the beginning of this chapter. The EMTs are doing CPR, everyone is rushing around, and once we get him inside, the man is "shocked" to bring his heart back to a normal rhythm. (We don't use paddles anymore like you see in the TV shows or do dramatic countdowns before we shock someone, but you get the picture.)

What most people don't know is that men in cardiac arrest are more likely to exhibit a pattern we call ventricular fibrillation, or V-fib. This is a type of cardiac arrhythmia in which the heart "quivers" rather than beats, resulting in loss of consciousness and little or no pulse. V-fib is also the "shockable" heart rhythm, meaning that an electrical jolt to the heart muscle will often "reset" the electrical impulses that control the ventricles and start the heart beating normally again.

One study found that if you're able to get the heart to restart in a case of V-fib, cooling the patient helps reduce inflammation and protects the brain during the healing process.[19] The idea is that you can live a lot longer when you're hypothermic than you can when you're overheating; the colder it is, the less energy your body uses on metabolic functions. So when we cool V-fib patients by way of cooling pads placed around the body or an intravenous device, they are more likely to wake up with their brain and other vital organs undamaged (or less damaged) by the short-term lack of blood flow.

Of course, this was a hugely exciting discovery, and hospitals around the country immediately began to put this simple cooling procedure into practice. But immediately, I noticed a big issue. The study was *only* performed on V-fib patients—who happen to be mostly men.

Women in cardiac arrest are more likely to come in with pulseless electrical activity (PEA), or asystole, which is where the heart stops beating altogether and "flatlines." And despite what happens on the TV dramas, this condition is not shockable. Unless the heart spontaneously restarts on its own (which does happen on occasion), our only tools are epinephrine and old-fashioned CPR.

This is just one example of how our male-centric approach creates innovative treatment options for men but underserves women. The fact is that V-fib patients have a better prognosis, so from a study-design standpoint, they were a better choice than patients with PEA to evaluate for this kind of neurological protection. Clinically and ethically, it makes sense to study the issue where you might be able to make a bigger difference; it's good study design.

The issue isn't that researchers chose to study V-fib. It's that, despite the enormous lifesaving implications of this research, women were underrepresented in it due to the nature of the condition being studied. In practice, research like this expands my options for treating V-fib patients but doesn't give me additional tools for treating many of my female cardiac arrest patients, because techniques like the one described above were not sanctioned for use in non-V-fib patients.

One current study is looking at cooling "non-shockables," which would solve a large portion of the issue mentioned above— but the results are years away from becoming part of the algorithm for treating PEA patients in ED settings. This kind of thing is fairly common. Studies are structured around male models first, and then "follow-up" studies look at the same treatments, procedures, or effects in women. But while those secondary studies are being approved and conducted, women lose out on potentially lifesaving benefits.

Then there's the issue of plain old exclusion. As I mentioned in Chapter 2, when we explored the evolution of male-centric medicine, women of reproductive age must often be tested for pregnancy as a condition of their participation in clinical trials, and there's always the concern that they might become pregnant during the course of the trial.[20] Recently, an ED physician and researcher invited to speak at Brown University outright admitted to me that his hospital had excluded female patients from their ED-based study because they didn't want to incur the time and expense of pregnancy testing. This underscores the reality that, in some clinical environments, female bodies are considered obstacles to effective research, not necessary factors in studying the human population.

Stroke: The Other Killer

Stroke, like heart disease, is a deadly condition related to blood flow—only here, we're looking at blood flow to the brain rather than to the heart.

Just as with heart disease, women have their own risk factors and presentation for stroke, few of which overlap with the male model. During a stroke, men often suffer a sudden loss of function on one side of the body. They may have drooping eyelids, garbled speech, and numbness—all the things we traditionally associate with stroke. Women, on the other hand, may have a headache akin to a migraine or a sudden change in mental or emotional status—and unless their providers know what to look for, they can be misdiagnosed or not diagnosed at all.

A great example of this happened in the ED recently. Often, during a shift change, the incoming staff have the opportunity to evaluate patients who haven't been formally diagnosed or discharged to other parts of the hospital. Earlier in the day, before I arrived, an elderly woman, whose nickname was Birdie, had been sent in by her nursing home. She'd had some mental-status changes that morning, was complaining of a headache, and had been struggling with her hand coordination. The nursing home staff thought she might have a urinary tract infection (UTI), which often causes mental-status changes and is common in elderly women. Her urine had been sent for analysis, but the test results weren't back yet.

"Have you considered stroke?" I asked the outgoing staff.

"But she just has a headache," someone replied—as if that excluded a stroke diagnosis.

Birdie's urinalysis came back normal, so my team went back to examine her a second time. We called the neurologist and ordered an MRI. The images indicated that Birdie did, in fact, have signs of stroke.

Stroke is the third-leading killer of women in the United States today. It kills twice as many women as breast cancer! In the U.K., stroke is the fourth largest cause of death among the general population, and although men have a greater chance of stroke, women are more likely to die as a result. However, the unique manifestations of stroke in women have only recently been discovered, and many physicians still do not understand the differences in risk and symptoms when assessing men and women. Therefore, stroke is often misdiagnosed—as it almost was for Birdie.

For example, men are slightly more likely than women to have transient ischemic attack (TIA), meaning small strokes with symptoms that go away after a few minutes, hours, or days, which are often hard to diagnose after they recede. However, more than half of all stroke deaths occur in women.

I believe that this could be partially related to the fact that TIA symptoms may be described differently by women than men.

If part of the brain is not getting blood and that part of the brain is only responsible for a small part of the body or a particular cognitive function, the symptoms may not seem "stroke-like." Women will come in with complaints like, "This weird thing happened today. I talked funny for five minutes, but now I'm fine." Or "I had total brain fog for an hour today, but everything seems okay now." When we look for evidence of a blood clot or impaired blood flow in the brain, we can't find anything, because the blood clot has already dissolved. This makes TIA extremely difficult to diagnose but also contributes to the subjective perception that women are more likely to exaggerate symptoms.

Because of situations like these, women's strokes are often misdiagnosed, brushed off, or mistaken for other common ailments, including UTIs, migraine, and—yes, you guessed it—anxiety. This can lead to a potentially deadly delay in treatment.

In general, a fear of adverse effects in women seems to pervade the medical mentality, and this affects how women are treated for stroke. For example, one study that looked at prescription of the anticoagulant dabigatran found that women were generally prescribed a lower dose, despite the fact that prescribing guidelines were the same for both men and women. Men were more likely to be given the recommended 150 mg dose for blood clot and stroke prevention, while women were more likely to receive the lower 110 mg dose.[21] Women had consistently poorer outcomes on this drug—unless they were prescribed the standard 150 mg dose, at which point their results improved. When asked why they chose the lower dose for women, many prescribers cited the greater chance of women falling down and injuring themselves as a reason to give less of the anticoagulant (since any cuts or injuries could result in excessive bleeding while on this medication), despite the fact that they had no data to back up this assertion. Thus, the perception among doctors that women were more likely to fall led to routine underprescribing of a lifesaving drug.

This is indicative of a broader problem, which is the perception that women are inherently weaker than men and need to be protected. We'll discuss this unconscious bias in more depth in Chapter 8, but it applies here in the sense that women routinely have to try far harder to get the right care and then are expected to apologize for continuing to seek the care they need when they don't receive it on the first, second, or third try.

The best thing that women can do is to know their risk factors. For example, migraine with aura is a risk factor for ischemic stroke, and as many as 70 percent of migraine sufferers are women. Other risk factors include high blood pressure, using birth control pills or other synthetic hormones, and pregnancy.[22] African American women are twice as likely to have a stroke as white women of the same age; this is due to several factors, including sickle-cell anemia (the most common genetic disorder in African Americans) and the fact that black women tend to have higher rates of high blood pressure, obesity, and diabetes.[23]

It's also vital for women to know the female-specific symptoms of stroke. A standard Google search for "stroke symptoms" will produce multiple images of men having strokes but little about women's presentation. A prospective, observational study presented at the American Stroke Association International Stroke Conference noted that "women were 43% more likely to report non-traditional stroke symptoms such as pain, changes in mental status, lightheadedness, headache, or other neurological and non-neurological symptoms."[24]

Therefore, women need to be aware that any or all of the following symptoms could indicate stroke:

- Loss of consciousness/fainting
- General weakness
- Shortness of breath or difficulty breathing
- Confusion, disorientation, or unresponsiveness
- Sudden behavioral changes or changes in mental status
- Agitation
- Nausea or vomiting

- Hiccups
- Headache
- Pain, including neck pain or pain in the extremities
- Seizures

As you can see, the symptoms of stroke in women often overlap with other conditions. This creates lack of recognition, which in turn results in delayed treatment and poorer outcomes. However, the most effective treatments for stroke—like the clot-busting drug tPA—are only available if the stroke is recognized and diagnosed early; otherwise, irreversible damage to the brain or blood vessels may occur. My colleague Tracy Madsen, MD, associate director of the Division of Sex and Gender in Emergency Medicine at Brown University's Department of Emergency Medicine and one of the country's leading researchers of sex differences in stroke, led a study that filled a critical knowledge gap in this area. In "Analysis of Tissue Plasminogen Activator Eligibility by Sex in the Greater Cincinnati/Northern Kentucky Stroke Study," Madsen et al. proved that although there are some small differences in individual tPA exclusion criteria, overall, women and men have similar eligibility for use of this lifesaving drug.[25]

This raises the question, *If criteria for tPA use are similar for women and men, why did a review study published by the* Journal of the American Heart Association *find that women were 30 percent less likely to receive tPA than their male counterparts?*[26] In that study, researchers Matthew Reeves, PhD, et al. concluded, "Despite the presence of significant between-study variation, women with acute stroke were consistently less likely to receive thrombolysis treatment compared with men. Further studies to explore the origins of this sex disparity are warranted."

Dr. Madsen's evidence suggests that any disparities in the use of tPA are potentially related to biases in care—including delayed recognition due to lack of information about female-pattern stroke. Such bias might contribute to other issues as well—such as why women have consistently worse recovery times after stroke than men and why they are more likely to live in a long-term health-care facility after a stroke event.

To me, all of this information fits into a pattern.

1. Women have worse outcomes in this area, including heart attack and stroke. Why? →

2. Do both men and women get the same treatments? No? →

3. Why don't men and women receive the same treatments? Is it because they are not eligible for those treatments? Did they undergo the same diagnostic tests? No? →

4. Do healthcare providers recognize the same disease in women as they do in men? Do women present differently? Yes? →

5. Why do women present differently? Is it because of an actual physical difference in disease pathology or because of a gender or cultural norm?

We should be asking this series of questions every time we are asked to diagnose or treat a woman.

My research division studies these patterns. We try to work backward to find the root cause and ultimately make a change in the foundational educational materials and treatment protocols for the condition. There's no question that women *are* biologically different and unique; we need to keep digging up all the areas where this difference is at play and adjust our conclusions accordingly.

Taking It Home

As women, we are so knowledgeable about our reproductive organs—about the obvious things that make us female. This is wonderful, but it's not enough to get a full picture of our health, especially when it comes to mortality rates and quality-of-life out-comes among women. Our health depends on knowing the truth about the real killers of women, including heart attack and stroke, and learning to recognize them even when—*especially* when—they don't present in accordance with textbook male symptom patterns.

The best way to apply the knowledge from this chapter in your life and the lives of your loved ones is to use your intuition, your powers of deduction, and your common sense. Despite all our knowledge as doctors, we can't actually feel or sense what you can feel and sense in your own body. We can't have the same experi-ence of your symptoms.

If you have symptoms congruent with heart disease or stroke/TIA, and you don't have the "traditional" risk factors for those con-ditions, you may be given a different diagnosis by default—just like Birdie or like Julie in Chapter 1. If so, the following may help you navigate your care in order to get the support you need:

- If you have any doubts or sense that something is wrong, in the case of heart disease or stroke, beyond what's been ex-plained to you, start a conversation with your provider. You might ask, "What criteria are you basing that diagnosis on?"

If the response is that you don't have hypertension, aren't a smoker, and don't have high cholesterol, you might reply, "But I do have these other risk factors that are specific to women." You might mention the preeclampsia that necessitated an induction in your second pregnancy or the inflammatory condition that increases your risk of microvascular disease.

- Express your concerns about the current diagnosis and why you think you may be dealing with a cardiovascular or neurovascular issue—even if those concerns are based mostly on your own gut feeling. This will open the doors to additional conversations, testing, and observation—and, ultimately, help you get the support and treatment you need and deserve.

- If you are at risk for or have symptoms congruent with microvascular dysfunction, you can also request a specialized stress test (if your hospital facility is able to provide one).

- Also, be very clear with your provider about what medications you are taking, particularly if you are using birth control pills, have a hormonal implant, or have an intrauterine device (IUD). So many women who come into the ED say no when asked if they take medication, but because hormones raise the risk of blood clotting, they are a genuine concern when it comes to heart and brain health. (We'll talk more about the role hormones play in our health in Chapter 6.)

What Matters—Your Key Takeaways

- Heart attack and stroke are not "men's" diseases. They are, respectively, the number one and number three killers of women in the United States today. In the U.K. more than twice as many women die each year from coronary heart disease than die from breast cancer.

- The symptoms and indicators of female-pattern heart attack and stroke may be very different from those for men. Knowing what female-patterns symptoms look like is vital to getting a timely diagnosis and treatment.

- Women are more likely to have "diffuse" disease, such as microvascular dysfunction, rather than the standard "blocked arteries" that we see in men. This makes it difficult for standard tests to pinpoint women's heart disease. Also, women with cardiac issues are more likely to be misdiagnosed than men.

- Both heart attack and stroke carry unique female risk factors. Among these are the use of exogenous hormones such as birth control pills and IUDs, pregnancy and postpartum complications, migraine, and inflammatory disorders.

- When talking to your provider about your symptoms, always be clear and share as much detail as possible.

chapter four

DRUGS FOR DIFFERENT BODIES: THE FEMALE SIDE OF PHARMACEUTICALS

Maria-Rosa was a robust woman in her late forties with a loud voice and an infectious laugh. She was a project manager at a local contracting firm, a grandmother, and a born nurturer. During her multiple visits to the emergency department, she got to know some of the staff and was constantly asking after their little ones and offering them her brand of "take-no-prisoners" life advice.

Every time we saw Maria-Rosa, it seemed to be for a different concern. The first few times, she came in with acute back pain. No matter what she did, the pain kept getting worse. Her diagnoses were inconclusive. Her surgery for spinal stenosis was not effective. The only solution we and her other doctors could offer was to keep ramping up her pain meds and recommend that she incorporate lifestyle adjustments like a healthy diet and gentle yoga. Eventually, the pain was so bad that she was prescribed oxycodone supplemented with ibuprofen between doses. Even then, she continued to visit the ED when the pain overwhelmed her and she couldn't safely take any more painkillers. We were able to arrange steroid injections and offer short-term IV pain meds but ultimately had to send her home without a lasting solution.

Understandably, Maria-Rosa's sleep was affected by her back pain. She couldn't get comfortable and woke up multiple times per night. Her constant fatigue began to affect her work. Her primary physician gave her Benadryl and Ambien to help her sleep.

Living with that level of pain and the resulting sleep disruptions also affected Maria-Rosa's mental state. She reported feeling anxious. Her therapist recommended antianxiety medication.

Then Maria-Rosa came into the ED with a raging urinary tract infection (UTI). The attending physician gave her Cipro, a powerful antibiotic, to kill the infection before it spread to her kidneys and made things even worse.

The last time I saw Maria-Rosa, she was on a stretcher, surrounded by frantic nurses and interns who were trying, without success, to restart her heart through CPR. According to her daughter, who'd made the call to 911, Maria-Rosa had been feeling "a little off all day, but it's nothing to worry about"—and then, while cooking dinner for her daughter and grandkids, she collapsed.

What happened to Maria-Rosa? How had idiopathic back pain—however excruciating—led to sudden cardiac death?

Multiple Drugs Multiply Risk

Maria-Rosa experienced, and ultimately died as a result of, an issue that is more common than many physicians would like to admit.

This issue isn't talked about much, but it is widespread. The average American adult takes four or more different prescriptions. Women are statistically more likely to be prescribed medications than men and are more likely to have prescriptions from multiple providers (who may or may not be aware of what other drugs the patient is taking, since most of this information is self-reported).[1] Furthermore, women are more likely to have adverse reactions or interactions since most drugs are tested primarily (or even exclusively) in men.

In Maria-Rosa's case, it's almost certain that her prescriptions, in combination, caused her ventricular tachycardia and ultimate sudden cardiac death.

Unfortunately, cases like hers happen all the time. Arrhythmia (when the heart does not beat normally) is often a *direct result* of drug interactions. When women's QT intervals (aka, the "resting time" between a person's heartbeats) are affected by various prescription drugs, the results can range from simple arrhythmia, to ventricular tachycardia (torsades de pointes), to asystole (flatline) and sudden cardiac death.

Before Maria-Rosa's back pain sent her into a "treatment spiral," her heart appeared perfectly healthy. So how could this happen? Shouldn't her doctors have known that the combination of her pain meds, antianxiety pills, steroids, and antibiotics were creating a deadly cocktail?

Perhaps they should have. But they didn't, because if Maria-Rosa had been a man, such a combination would likely not have produced the same effect—or *even been dangerous at all*.

The key to understanding this deadly disparity lies in the QT interval. Men have shorter QT intervals than women; this is a result of the surge in testosterone that occurs during male puberty.

In short, men's hearts need less time to recover between contractions (i.e., heartbeats) than women's do.

Many prescription drugs—such as painkillers, anti-inflammatory drugs, steroids, sleep aids, antibiotics, antihistamines, and antidepressants, to name a few—have the effect of incrementally increasing a person's QT interval. When such drugs are taken alone, this usually isn't cause for concern, as the effect is minimal. However, when such drugs are taken in combination over a period, the QT interval is increased to the point where the heart doesn't beat correctly after its elongated rest period. When this tipping point is reached, the heart just... sputters out. This is called "drug-induced torsades de pointes," and it's more common in women than in men—precisely because women lack the testosterone-protective effect and end up taking more prescription medications then men. In fact a German study found that, between 2008 and 2011, the majority (66 percent) of "long QT syndrome" patients were female and that 60 percent of those female cases were confirmed as drug-related according to World Health Organization criteria.[2]

In Maria-Rosa's case, it was the antibiotics that put her over that QT interval tipping point. But for millions of other women around the country, it could be that new antidepressant, that new immunosuppressant for fibromyalgia, or even an extra daily dose of over-the-counter antacid.

Because her doctors outside the ED may have been unaware of female sex as an independent risk factor for serious drug interactions, because women are more likely to have multiple or overlapping providers and prescribers (with each provider potentially unaware of existing prescriptions unless the patient reports them), and because our current system isn't set up to take QT interval into account when prescribing new drugs, Maria-Rosa wasn't offered the tests and alternatives that could have prevented her death. Even though my emergency department is at the cutting edge of sex and gender medicine, it isn't a routine part of our protocol to check a woman's QT interval before prescribing a simple round of antibiotics for a UTI.

We need to do better.

Metabolism Doesn't Just Apply to Food

The QT interval issue is only one of hundreds of disparities between men's and women's physiology, but it serves to illustrate just how deadly these disparities can be. In addition to this crucial area of heart functioning, women also exhibit unique attributes in the areas of bone structure and composition, body fat composition and location, tissue elasticity, and neurological function, to name a few.

Another huge difference between men and women is the way they process various compounds in their bodies. These sex-based differences mean that pharmaceuticals are digested, processed, and distributed differently in women's systems and that women experience more unanticipated side effects from taking prescription drugs than men.

These differences were highlighted in a 2014 article by Theresa Chu, PhD, in the journal *U.S. Pharmacist*. She wrote, "Sex differences in metabolism (phase I and II) are believed to be the major cause of differential pharmacokinetics [responses to pharmaceuticals in the body] between men and women. Many CYP450 enzymes (phase I metabolism) show a sex-dependent difference in activity. Most of the phase II enzymes have a higher activity in men than in women.... Sex differences are also found in other pharmacokinetic parameters such as drug absorption, drug distribution, and excretion. Despite these differences between men and women, sex-specific dosing recommendations are absent for most drugs."[3] While that may seem like a lot to digest, the key takeaway is the final line.

Here's one example of these metabolic differences at work in an unexpected place:

We've all heard that women metabolize alcohol differently than men. It's recommended that women only have one alcoholic drink per day, while men can have two. And it takes only half as much alcohol to get a woman drunk as it does a man.

The reason for this is an enzyme called aldehyde dehydrogenase (ADH). Men have a lot of this enzyme—in men, ADH is present in both the stomach lining and in the liver—and it's very active. Women, on the other hand, have little to no ADH in the stomach lining, and it is less active in the liver. This means that men begin to metabolize alcohol immediately after they consume it and that much of it is digested before it ever gets into the bloodstream. In women, however, the alcohol must enter the bloodstream in order for the liver to secrete ADH, and so digestion is both slower and less efficient. Body fat percentage and distribution also appear to play a role; the higher a person's body fat percentage, the higher his or her blood alcohol content after the same number of drinks.[4] In general, women tend to have higher body fat percentages than men.

The result of these sex-based metabolic differences is that a man and a woman of the same height, weight, and age can consume the same amount of alcohol, but the woman will feel the effects sooner and more strongly, and after three drinks her blood alcohol level will be 25 percent higher than that of a man.

I remember learning about this many years ago in medical school; it was one of many, many facts flung at us to memorize and learn in one of our conference hall sessions. This fact stuck out to me, though. It made me wonder, *Oh? Men and women are different? Why?* But then, we were moving on to a different set of facts and figures, and my question receded.

Later, I saw this fact used in public health bulletins; my friends' kids learned it in high school health classes. But there are concerns at play here beyond the public health implications of higher rates of alcohol poisoning and intoxication-related injuries in women. After all, our bodies didn't evolve to produce ADH simply to digest booze!

As it turns out, multiple medications and compounds are broken down, at least in part, by aldehyde dehydrogenase—including the highly popular sleep aid Ambien (zolpidem).

Women metabolize Ambien differently than men for the same reasons that they metabolize alcohol differently. The breakdown of Ambien likely begins for men in the stomach; for women, in the bloodstream. (While studies have shown that ADH is at play in Ambien metabolism, there are likely many other enzymes that play a role, many of which may be sex differentiated.) The result of this difference in metabolic process is that the morning after women take the drug, their serum concentrations are nearly twice those of men—which results in grogginess, "brain fog," and (for some) physical impairment equivalent to alcohol intoxication.

This is not acceptable. Women have busy lives, and many take sleep aids so that they can continue to function at the levels demanded of them by their many responsibilities. Because researchers didn't understand that small differences in metabolic function between men and women can have big consequences, women were basically waking up and moving through the day impaired. In fact, some of the studies conducted around this were driving simulations; both in the lab and in real life, the driving of women on Ambien resembled that of an intoxicated person. We still don't know exactly how many auto accident deaths and injuries have resulted from women using Ambien at the higher dose based on male physiology, but the number is not small.

Unfortunately, but also not unpredictably, this phenomenon was not discovered until many years after the drug's release, when government monitors noticed that the vast majority of complaints regarding Ambien were filed by women or their doctors, all reporting similar side effects. This difference in rates of metabolism and serum concentrations was not considered significant in the initial drug trials (even though those trials did demonstrate that women had higher serum concentrations than men) because the researchers did not deem sex differences significant and did not differentiate adverse reactions by sex in their final findings. Male-dominated future studies (including those used to produce generic variations) did not capture this issue either.

But here's the thing: even twenty years ago, when the drug was released, we had all the pertinent information; we knew that ADH levels in women affect the way they process certain compounds. Did drug researchers know that Ambien was broken down by ADH at the time of its release? I can't say. But the fact is, no one put two and two together until thousands of women came forward to complain about their side effects.

Ambien is not an isolated case. In fact, a 2001 report from the Government Accountability Organization found that, out of ten prescription drugs withdrawn from the market from 1997 to 2001, eight were found to pose greater health risks for women.[5] Worse, one-third of those "greater health risks" were for torsades de pointes—meaning that the drugs were withdrawn after causing sudden cardiac death in women who were not otherwise considered at risk.

Hormones Impact Drug Metabolism

Metabolic differences between men and women aren't limited to enzymes. Women also process drugs differently during different phases of their menstrual cycles.

This means that serum levels of vital drugs like Dilantin (phenytoin), a powerful anticonvulsant seizure medication, can dip dangerously low on certain days of the month. Women often have breakthrough seizures during times of hormonal fluctuation, sometimes resulting in serious physical injuries from falls or automobile accidents.

Drug-related QT interval prolongation is also affected by the menstrual cycle. At certain points of the cycle, some drugs have been shown to cause a greater increase in the length of the QT interval. If a premenopausal patient is on multiple QT-prolonging drugs, she could therefore be at far greater risk of asystole or other cardiac events during certain days of her cycle.

While it's clear that women's menstrual cycles do have a measurable and potentially damaging impact on drug metabolism, there are few guidelines or even suggestions to help prescribers address this. While there is information out there about how certain classes of medication (some HIV meds, antiseizure meds, antidepressants, benzodiazepines, and one class of antibiotics) might render birth control less effective, I have not found any alternate dosing formulas to balance those few days when serum levels are impacted by hormone spikes or drops. Often, the possibility of premenstrual breakthrough incidents or QT prolongation isn't even discussed when the drug is prescribed—and these potential complications are rarely, if ever, considered in an emergency setting. Women are taken completely by surprise.

The flip side of this discussion is how hormones themselves are affected by drugs—particularly when prescribed hormones, like birth control pills, are in use.

A woman came into the ED recently with a case of "vaginal bleeding and anxiety" (according to her triage assessment). Of course, whenever I hear "anxiety" coupled with a female issue my ears perk up. There was more to this story, I knew.

Turns out, the woman, whose name was Saira, had gone to her doctor several months ago because of recurring migraine headaches. She was prescribed topiramate, which is effective for migraines but also interferes with the efficacy of oral birth control. Her prescriber did not mention this to her.

A month later, Saira was pregnant. She and her husband decided that they were not in a position—financially or otherwise—to expand their family, so she went to her local clinic and received medication to assist with an abortion. After suffering through several days of heavy bleeding and intense cramping, she thought the worst was over—until, about four weeks later, when the intense cramps and vaginal bleeding started again.

Saira didn't have "anxiety." She was in pain and scared. After I ordered an ultrasound, it was clear that she needed an emergency dilatation and curettage (D&C) to remove what we call "retained products of conception." Had she not come to the ED, she might have suffered serious effects—including systemic infection, hemorrhage, or even the loss of the ability to bear children in the future.

Saira lost several days of work because of her symptoms. She had to be admitted to the hospital for the D&C, as it had to be conducted under general anesthesia (which carries its own risks); this meant more time out of work and finding care for her other three children so that her husband didn't lose days of necessary income as well.

All these layers of risk and impact—to her health, her family, and her financial situation—could have been avoided if Saira's provider had simply informed her that her migraine medication would impact her birth control. To me, this is just another indication that we need to place greater value on women's reproductive rights across the board in medicine. Since 17 percent of women of reproductive age in the United States are currently using oral birth control (versus only 10 percent using condoms),[6] it's imperative that we both understand and share with women how certain drugs can affect the efficacy of birth control and vice versa—how birth control can affect the performance of other drugs.

We'll talk more about pharmaceutical hormones in Chapter 7, but for now, it's important to know that the ways in which drugs—including hormones—combine in a woman's body can produce complications that don't have any equivalents in the male model.

Our Drug-Testing Protocol Ignores Sex Differences

Drug companies, both in the U.S. and worldwide, attempting to remedy this gap by including greater percentages of women in their phase III studies (larger human trials). In fact, a 2009 analysis found that 6 to 7 percent of new drug applications that included a sex analysis showed *at least* a 40 percent difference in pharmacokinetics (the movement of drugs inside the body) between men and women.[7] Basically, this shows us that we barely look for these kinds of differences in our study design—but when we do, we see that women metabolize drugs differently than men more than 40 percent of the time.

Despite this overwhelming evidence of the necessity of such research, in the vast majority of drug trials, women and men are *not* analyzed separately according to sex-based criteria. When studies are designed without such criteria, the different effects of the drugs on men and women often simply cancel each other out. For example, men may have no increase in QT interval with a particular drug, whereas women may have a large, dangerous increase. When these results are lumped together by researchers, it results in a statistically insignificant QT interval impact, which the Food and Drug Administration (FDA) then deems an "acceptable risk" when it reviews the study in the process of drug approval.

The norms for preclinical testing of pharmaceuticals are also set up to favor male-centric outcomes. In 76 percent of cases, researchers don't even know the sex of the cells they're working with in their tests. As we've learned, male cells can operate differently from female cells both individually and cooperatively, owing to the differences in gene expression. When something works in the petri dish in the lab according to the male (XY) chromosome paradigm, there's no guarantee it will perform the same way in the female (XX) cells. And yet, male-centric testing models persist.

As "bench to bedside" research proceeds, the drug moves into animal testing. Around 80 percent of animals used in pharmaceutical testing are healthy young males.

By the time a drug reaches human clinical trials, it's been "proven" to have baseline efficacy and safety in male cells and on male animals. In the past, when researchers did bring women into the equation, they weren't looking for variables unique to the female physiology. In fact, those variables may not even have been included in the study model, even if women were sprinkled into the mix of study participants. Instead, researchers were looking for manifestations of adverse effects observed in the previous *male* subjects. These were the observations that were ultimately collated and submitted to the FDA pending final approval for the public.

You can see how easy it has been historically for a product like Ambien to make its way onto the market without anyone knowing how seriously our ignorance of sex differences and dosing requirements could impact women. Things are improving now that we are starting to understand sex differences, but change is slow. According to a recent FDA report, women's participation in phase I trials—the phase where factors like initial efficacy and dosage, and dose toleration are determined—is still only around 30 percent.

So what happens when a drug that hasn't been extensively tested in women is still marketed to and prescribed for women? What is being done to protect women or warn them of potential unidentified adverse effects?

Frighteningly little, as it turns out.

The sheer number of adverse reactions reported with Ambien prompted government controllers to research the issue. The result was a recommendation that women be prescribed half doses to cancel out the differences in female metabolism of the compound. However, most of our current pharmaceutical repertoire— from pain relievers, to hypertensives, to immunosuppressants, to stomach acid blockers—were designed according to a male model and ultimately brought to human trials via a male-centric and male-focused testing model. The truth is, we simply *don't know* how many popular drugs affect women differently because, quite frankly, after-market studies are not a priority for pharmaceutical companies. Dr. Francis Collins, director of the National Institutes of Health, said in his TED talk that it takes upward of fourteen years and $1 billion to get a single new drug approved.[8] After all that, pharma companies have little incentive to pursue further studies that might force them to recall it!

In the U.S. the FDA does try to support evidence-gathering for drugs available to the public market. According to its website, "Despite The [Center for Drug Evaluation and Research's] vigilant premarket review, active post-marketing surveillance of drug adverse effects is also essential. In the U.K., the MHRA (Medical and Healthcare products Regulatory Authority) encourages doctors and patients to report adverse effects via the Yellow Card Scheme. Because all possible side effects of a drug can't be anticipated based on preapproval studies involving only several hundred to several thousand patients, FDA maintains a system of post-marketing surveillance and risk assessment programs to identify adverse events that did not appear during the drug approval process. FDA monitors adverse events such as adverse reactions and poisonings. The Agency uses this information to update drug labeling, and, on rare occasions, to reevaluate the approval or marketing decision." There are clear procedures in place for reporting adverse effects and for reviewing that reported data. (This is how the issues with women's metabolism of Ambien were discovered and the prescribing guidelines changed.)

Pharmaceutical companies are required to report any evidence presented to them about drug interactions, complications, and the like. Doctors, nurses, and other medical practitioners can report data directly. Also, consumers can report issues with drugs through the FDA Adverse Event Reporting System (FAERS) Public Dashboard.[9] This is a fantastic way for consumers to make their voices heard. Unfortunately, reporting such incidents after the fact doesn't help the patients who have already suffered adverse effects.

In my mind, changes in the way we study and approve premarket drugs will only come as the result of a massive public outcry. Performing sex-based analysis increases the cost of studies because you have to enroll more subjects and analyze them separately. However, the cost on the back end—both in human terms and in terms of the burden on our medical system—far outweighs any additional up-front investment. We have a moral and fiscal obligation to change our practices *now* and to demand testing based on sex throughout the process so that women don't suffer later.

Our Prescribing Guidelines Aren't Designed for Women

When I asked my colleague Barbara Roberts, MD—a prominent cardiologist and author of *The Truth About Statins: Risks and Alternatives to Cholesterol-Lowering Drugs*—about unnecessary prescriptions of popular drugs in women, she shared with me the following:

> There is zero evidence that primary prevention with statins in high-risk women lowers the risk of hard endpoints like heart attack, stroke or death. The JUPITER (Justification for the Use of Statins in Prevention: An Intervention Trial Evaluating Rosuvastatin) trial was said to show benefit in women, but that's only because they included the very soft end point of unstable chest pain syndromes. If you look at the hard endpoints, there was no benefit in women.
>
> In addition, women in the rosuvastatin group in JUPITER had an increased risk of developing diabetes. Even when you do a meta-analysis of statins for secondary prevention, the absolute risk reduction in women is only 3%, half of what it is in men.

> I concluded after many years of patient care that statins were very good at lowering LDL cholesterol but ineffective in lowering the risk of vascular events. LDL is a weak risk factor in men and not a risk factor in women at all unless HDL is low.[10]

Statins—cholesterol-lowering drugs like the popular brand Lipitor—are some of the most prescribed drugs in America right now. And yet, they appear to have little, if any, benefit for the millions of women taking them.

Once again, it comes back to the male-centric model.

High cholesterol does, in fact, appear to be a minor risk factor for heart attack in men. High levels of LDL ("bad" cholesterol) correspond, to some degree, to the levels of plaque buildup in male arteries. As we know, it is this plaque that causes blockages in the blood vessels, resulting in "traditional" heart attack patterns like myocardial infarction.

But studies are revealing that this is not the case for women. In fact, as Dr. Roberts shared, elevated LDL isn't a risk factor *at all* for women unless their HDL is also low.

So why are so many women taking statins every day?

Many would blame this on "Big Pharma" and its marketing tactics, and I'm sure that's true to some degree. (I recall a particular advertisement from years ago when Lipitor was supposed to be the "heart attack saver"; it showed an older, overweight man sitting next to a thin, thirty-something woman, showing them with identical cholesterol levels. Essentially, the implication was that everyone should be taking Lipitor for heart attack prevention.) But the underlying issue is the medical model that argues that if it's good for men, it's good for women. And since, as we learned in Chapter 3, sex differences are rarely accounted for in cardiac studies (or any research trials),[11] the evidence would seem to bear out this false assumption.

Most of the most popular drugs on the market have not been tested specifically in or for women. For instance, Lisinopril (a type of antihypertensive in a class called ACE inhibitors and currently the most prescribed drug in America) is known to "reduce fetal renal function and increase fetal and neonatal morbidity and death" in the second and third trimesters of pregnancy.[12] However, we have little information about how this drug affects women of childbearing age who are not pregnant and whether its use causes complications in later pregnancies even if the drug is discontinued. At this point, women are simply taken off Lisinopril and put on one of a number of different blood pressure medications—which may or may not have been studied in pregnant women. (A recent Canadian study found that only 43 percent of trials of ACE inhibitors reported any sex-specific outcomes at all.)[13]

Seemingly benign drugs can also be contraindicated for women. For example, it's common knowledge that low-dose aspirin therapy is helpful to reduce the risk of a first heart attack because aspirin acts as a blood thinner and anticlotting agent. However, that benefit has been observed *only* in men. In women, the reduced risk of a first heart attack from aspirin therapy did not outweigh the increased risk of gastrointestinal bleeding, ulcers, and other bleeding disorders. Yet so many women and their doctors assume, once again, that because aspirin therapy is helpful for men, it must also be helpful and safe for women.

And sometimes drugs that are lifesaving for men can be life-destroying for women. In a study published in the *Journal of Substance Abuse Treatment*, both men and women were given high-dose naltrexone, an antiaddiction drug often used worldwide, in addition to traditional psychotherapy, to treat patients with cocaine and alcohol addictions. Researchers found that "150mg/day of naltrexone added to a psychosocial treatment resulted in reductions in cocaine and alcohol use, and drug severity in men, compared to higher rates of cocaine and alcohol use and drug severity in women."[14] In other words, the drug—an opioid receptor antagonist that inhibits the feeling of euphoria associated with alcohol and drug use, rendering the user less likely to abuse these substances—reduced the use of alcohol and drugs in men but actually *increased* it in women, leading to a greater incidence of overdose, drug-related injury, and other complications. There was also evidence that women were more susceptible to common side effects of the medication, such as nausea and vomiting.

We don't yet know why this dose of naltrexone doesn't work for many women. Is it that alcohol and drugs work on different receptors for women? Is it that women are more likely to drink and use drugs to self-medicate for depression and anxiety, while men are more likely to seek a "high"? Is it that women metabolize naltrexone differently and so are not reaping the same physiological benefits of the drug as men?

What is most troubling to me is not the number of questions we have but the fact that these differences are not being taken into account when therapies and treatments are designed.

More, the findings of studies like the above are not filtering into the educational literature we provide to our medical students. Not long ago, I presented on sex differences to a group of female doctors and students in New York City. When I mentioned naltrexone, one of the students raised her hand, looking stricken.

"I just learned about this, and no one told me to consider the sex of the patient when prescribing naltrexone," she said. "I had a woman with severe alcohol addiction in my family medicine rotation a couple of months ago. She'd been picked up on the side of the road and brought to the ED where they saved her life. After she was discharged from the hospital, she followed up with us in the clinic. My attending physician and I gave her naltrexone because it looked like the best option out of the four drugs actually approved to treat alcohol abuse. Less than a month later, she came in again, same issue. She was almost dead. Again. I didn't understand why the meds weren't helping her stop drinking and doing drugs!"

I answered, "This is why we need woman-specific information and research. Some drugs, like naltrexone, may have different effects on women compared to men. Others, we just have no idea. It's important to consider these differences as they may, quite literally, mean the difference between life and death."

Every time I prescribe a drug in the ED, I ask myself, *What is the biological sex of the patient? Do I need to prescribe a lower dose (e.g., Ambien) or a higher dose (e.g., propofol)? Are there any female-specific side effects? How is this drug affected by the menstrual cycle? What is the woman's pregnancy history, and how might that affect her risks for cardiac and other conditions?* And if we don't have any research one way or the other, I ask, *Do the benefits outweigh the potential risks?* In other words, I need to do a woman-specific evaluation over and above our existing prescribing guidelines.

To those of us who know the difference, this has simply become part of our process when working with patients. But I also know that this is, in part, because sex and gender medicine is my focus. For most physicians, a good portion of what we learned in medical school is now irrelevant, outdated, or overwritten—particularly with regard to sex differences. My hope is that, as more data regarding sex-based and personalized medicine comes to light, doctors and other practitioners will be supported educationally and procedurally to do this type of "matching" in everyday clinical settings. But for now, it's up to both the individual doctors and their patients to ask the right questions and employ critical thinking to find the right solutions.

A Generic Problem

There's another major component of the pharmaceutical system that disproportionately affects women, and that is generic medications.

Over 80 percent of drugs prescribed in the United States are generic brands. Ostensibly, this keeps costs down for both patients and providers, but it also leads women even deeper into uncharted territory. Why? Because generic drugs are tested almost exclusively on young, healthy males. More, while their key chemical components may be identical to those of brand-name drugs, the additives and fillers used may be quite different. For women, this often means that generic drugs aren't absorbed as well as brand-name drugs or that they have unforeseen side effects.

Because the "active ingredient" of a generic is already approved for use in patients (due to the trials undergone to gain approval for the brand-name version of the drug), generic companies are only required to conduct something called "bioequivalence testing." This means that they need to prove that their generic version of the drug exhibits similar peak concentration and other effects in the body. Generic companies also get a 20 percent "fudge factor," meaning that they need to prove between 80 to 120 percent bioequivalence to the brand-name drug in order to bring a generic to market. These studies are conducted almost exclusively in young, healthy males, often over a period of just a few weeks. If bioequivalence can be proven, the generic is ready to be sold to the public.

Generic companies don't feel that they need to use women in their testing process because all they're doing is a "crossover" study design, checking for this bioequivalency. And since the false assumption that what's good for men is good for women is still so pervasive in medical research, it's considered perfectly acceptable to give a generic drug to a group of healthy men for two weeks; check their peak serum concentrations, absorption, and elimination stats (collectively called AUC, or "area under the curve," referring to how the information looks when plotted on a graph); and declare the generic medically comparable to its brand-name cousin.

It sounds simple, but for women, the reality of generics is far more complex.

The issues around how generics affect women aren't just due to the "active ingredients" of the drugs, because those are actually equivalent to brand-name versions. (Of course, the primary components may also never have been tested in women at all—there are situations where a cascade of male-centric testing has left us with little to no information about how the drug performs in women's bodies.) But the more insidious issue with generics is the "inactive ingredients," or fillers, which make up the bulk of the pill, capsule, liquid, or gelcap. In the medical world, we call these compounds "excipients."

These excipients can change the way a generic medication is absorbed and processed by the body—and they often create far different responses in women's bodies than in men's. For example, many generics use polyethylene glycol (PEG) as an excipient in their formulations. In studies of generic ranitidine (which is sold under the brand name Zantac), the use of PEG as a filler increased bioavailability by 63 percent. Researchers then concluded that they could use less of the active compound in their formulations and expect their product to produce equivalent results to its brand-name counterpart.

But here's the thing: PEG increased bioavailability in men, but it actually *decreased* it by 24 percent in women! So generic raniti-dine produced with PEG was actually only about half as effective for women as it was for men at an equivalent dose.

This isn't an isolated case. Some of the top generic medica-tions on the market (both over-the-counter and prescription) are formulated with PEG—including acetaminophen, escitalopram (brand name: Lexapro), and even oxycodone.

Several studies have found similar bioequivalence discrepan-cies between generics and brand-name drugs in women. A study by Mei-Ling Chen, PhD, et al. found that, out of twenty-three specific drug studies, there were statistically different results be-tween genders in five medications (22 percent) with respect to AUC variability.[15] In other words, the efficacy of these generics was greatly different in women than in the men in which the drugs had been studied.

A related review by Stuart MacLeod, PhD, et al. also asked this pointed question: "Compelling evidence has been presented to make the case that one cannot assume BE [bioequivalence] in women on the basis of studies conducted in men. So why does this practice continue? Why do regulatory agencies still accept results of BE in men for drugs to be used only by women?"[16]

Why, indeed?

As we've discussed, studying women is considered "problem-atic" by many medical researchers. Using only men in generic trials saves time and money. But in order to understand whether generics are actually bioequivalent for women, we need to conduct sex-specific studies that look at how these drugs react in women's bodies—especially important drugs like muscle relaxers, antibiotics, and pain relievers that we use all the time in hospital and clinical settings.

As you can see, the differences between generic and brand-name drugs are real and measurable. Unfortunately, however, when a woman shares with her doctor that the generic version of her prescription isn't working as well, or is causing gastrointestinal distress, or is simply making her "feel funny," her complaint will often be brushed off, because the general consensus in the medical world is still that generics are equivalent to brand-name drugs in every way because their bioequivalence has been "proven" in clinical research.

It's yet another manifestation of "it's all in her head." But the differences between generics and brand-name drugs are real, and so are their consequences for women.

Whenever a woman comes into the ED with breakthrough symptoms (like suddenly high blood pressure when she's already taking medication to control her hypertension), I often ask, "Did you switch to a generic recently?" Many times, a change in insurance status will encourage (or force) women to change to a less expensive variety of their medication; our hospital prescribing systems also default to generics over brand-name drugs in many cases.

Generics are important because they make necessary drugs more affordable. But when taking a generic means dealing with reduced efficacy or additional side effects, it's not a good trade-off. If you have noticed a difference in your symptoms since you started a generic medication or are noticing breakthrough events that weren't present when you were taking another version of your drug, your generic might be the problem.

Talk to your physician about finding a different generic version or returning to the brand-name version of your medication. Don't be afraid to bring this up; if you sense a difference in how you feel on your generic, chances are there are differences that could be impacting you!

Taking It Home

So, what can you do to make sure you aren't prescribed medications that are unnecessary, contraindicated, or downright dangerous for a female body?

The best thing to do is to be transparent with your providers, prescribers, and pharmacist. There are also several small, simple steps you can take to minimize your risk of drug interactions.

Because women are more likely than men to use multiple medications and have multiple prescribers, it's very important to do the following:

- Make a list of all of your medications, even the ones you don't think of as "drugs" (like birth control pills, vitamins, herbs, and over-the-counter medications like aspirin and ibuprofen), and carry this list with you at all times—not only to your doctors' appointments. (After all, no one ever plans to go to the ED!)
- Make sure that if you visit the hospital, all your new medications are "reconciled" with your old ones. Medication reconciliation (aka, Med Rec) is vital for patients because it can reveal discrepancies in dosing, drug interactions, and other concerns.

- Make sure that you leave the hospital with a complete list of everything you should be taking and any changes to your previous medications—including appropriate doses.
- Use the same pharmacy (or at least the same pharmacy chain) for all your medications.
- Try to work with one "umbrella" provider for all your medical concerns. Make sure this provider knows all the medications you're taking and in what doses. Review your prescription profile with this provider regularly.
- Ask your providers/prescribers if the drugs you're using have any special concerns, dosing guidelines, or contraindications for women.
- Next time you pick up a prescription, ask your pharmacist to review your medication profile to look for any possible interactions.
- Ask your providers/prescribers if any of your medications put you at risk for long QT syndrome—and if so, what your options are to reduce your risk of cardiac issues.
- Ask for an electrocardiogram to determine your current base-line QT time so that you can monitor your heart function if new drugs are added. This is particularly important if you are on known QT-prolonging agents. (And remember, even short-term prescriptions like antibiotics, antihistamines, or painkillers can dangerously elongate your QT interval.)
- Inform your providers/prescribers if you observe any adverse effects from your generic drugs. (There may be another generic that will work better for you.)
- Check with your prescriber or pharmacist before you add any over-the-counter remedies such as aspirin, ibuprofen, heartburn remedies (like Nexium or Prilosec), or antihistamines

to make sure that you are not putting yourself at risk for woman-specific side effects or interactions.

- Let your doctor know about any side effects you are experiencing from your medications, generic or otherwise, so they can add them to the FAERS (adverse drug reaction) database. (You can also add them yourself!)

- Above all, if you're not sure what a particular medication is for or if you truly need it, ask. The more knowledge you have, the better choices you can make for your health!

You can also do your own research, particularly with regard to whether your current medications have been evaluated in women. The FDA Drug Trials Snapshots website is a wonderful resource for discovering whether women were included in clinical trials for particular drugs, whether sex was considered as a variable, and whether particular side effects or dosing requirements have been noted for women. Many of my patients have used this.

While I don't advocate self-diagnosing via the internet, having a baseline understanding of your current prescriptions and how they might function in your female body is a great way to begin a conversation with your providers. As you've seen throughout this book, this sex-specific information isn't taught in medical school; doctors must do their own research. Therefore, you may find that your providers have varying levels of knowledge around this issue. Don't be afraid to start a conversation and ask questions.

Finally, if you are taking medications that are not proven to be effective in women, or if you are at risk for drug interactions because you are on multiple medications, don't just stop taking them; this may cause even bigger issues! Instead, talk to your provider about how you can reduce or eliminate your medications safely.

While many common diseases, like diabetes and heart disease, do have a genetic component, many are created or made worse by lifestyle factors. If you feel like your medications are jeopardizing your health, making small changes to your diet and exercise may be enough to lessen your pharmaceutical burden and help reduce your risk of drug-related complications.

The vast array of pharmaceuticals in our modern medical system is amazing. The drugs to which we have access routinely save lives and improve outcomes. Someday, I hope that we will have as much information about how drugs operate in women's bodies as we have about how they operate in men's. But until we have better testing of medications in women and better understanding of how drugs interact with one another and with the various complexities of the female body, we're in a bit of a Wild West situation. In the meantime, it's up to women to protect themselves through awareness and advocacy and by speaking up when they have questions.

Above all remember that you are not "silly" or "anxious" or "hysterical" because you have questions about how your prescriptions are affecting your body and its health. What you feel and sense is not "all in your head." Don't be afraid to ask the questions that will help you find the answers you need and the quality of care you deserve. After all, your inquiry might point your provider in the direction of a new discovery!

What Matters—Your Key Takeaways

- Long QT syndrome is a major contributor to cardiac events in women. Multiple medications increase the risk of QT elongation.

- Many prescription medications, including widely prescribed drugs like statins, antihypertensives, and over-the-counter medications may not be beneficial for women.

- Not all prescription drugs are studied in women. Often we don't learn about adverse effects in women until after the drug has been released to the general public.

- Generic drugs don't always function the same way as their brand-name counterparts. If you notice adverse effects from your generic prescription, it's not "all in your head." Talk to your provider about making a change.

- Always carry a list of all your prescription and over-the-counter medications so that you and your provider can make informed decisions when adding or changing medications.

chapter five

"HONEY, IT'S ALL IN YOUR HEAD": WOMEN'S INTUITION VERSUS WOMEN'S IMAGINATION

NOT LONG AGO, I was working an overnight shift in the emergency department when a woman named Lydia came in with flu-like symptoms and difficulty breathing.

Lydia was kind and funny but clearly exasperated. "I can't believe I'm here again," she sighed. "This place makes my skin crawl."

Despite being in significant discomfort and obviously exasperated, she was talkative. I had a lot of other patients to see, but her eyes captured me, and something made me pause. *I'm going to let her tell me her story*, I thought.

Turns out that when Lydia was forty years old, she was told that she needed a hysterectomy to deal with her uterine fibroids. Her ovaries and cervix were left intact. A few months later, at her follow-up, she asked her surgeon, "Why do I still have so much pain? It hurts even when I touch my stomach."

"Oh," the surgeon replied, "that's phantom uterus pain. Like when someone loses a limb and still feels it there."

"My uterus never hurt this much when I had one," Lydia snapped back. But the surgeon refused to examine her further.

Lydia went to several other specialists and finally found another surgeon who was willing to do an exploratory surgery—and eventually diagnosed her with stage-four endometriosis. That surgeon took out her cervix and fallopian tubes.

For months after the surgery, Lydia kept passing blood clots. Concerned, she went back to the surgeon. "The pain isn't gone," she told him. "And why the heck am I still bleeding?"

"That's normal," the surgeon assured her. "You're fine. Just take it easy."

Lydia knew there was more to it than that. She fought to have another exploratory surgery. Months later, she finally went back to the operating room—where her surgeon found a huge abscess infection on one of her ovaries. Now she needed to have her ovaries removed too.

As Lydia related this story to me, her eyes filled with tears. "I went through five years of hell," she said. "No one believed me. And then, I was *right*, but still no one believed me. They all treated me like I was stupid—like I couldn't possibly know that something was wrong with me. But it was real."

"I'm so sorry this happened to you," I told her. "We're trying to do better."

"You listened to me," she said, reaching over to pat my hand. "You're already doing better."

Lydia's story is a classic example of the ingrained bias that exists against women in the medical community. Every day, across all areas of medicine, in doctor's offices and emergency rooms around the country, women are told some variation of that patronizing statement:

"Honey, it's all in your head."

Let me be clear: this isn't only about feminism—although, as you know, I am a feminist. This isn't only about women's perception of how they are treated by doctors and providers. This is about a scientifically validated reality in the world of medicine. Women are being misdiagnosed, undertreated, and underserved, in part because providers don't believe them when they say something is wrong.

When we ask questions like, Why do women have overall poorer outcomes in major areas of health? or Why are women misdiagnosed so often? we need to look not only at women's unique biology (as we've done in the last several chapters) but at the societal conventions that play out in the collective unconscious around who women are and who they are not.

And as the mounting evidence shows, one thing is certain: women are *not* liars.

The Nature of Implicit Bias

My husband, who is also a physician, told me something recently that perfectly encapsulated how women's unique symptoms are often regarded (or rather, disregarded) in the medical field.

Apparently, a well-known (white, male) neurologist was speaking to one of my husband's colleagues in the break room of the hospital.

"You know we have an algorithm for paresthesia," he began.

Paresthesia is the medical term for "pins and needles." It can signify the onset of multiple sclerosis or Bell's palsy from Lyme disease. It's not painful, but it's pronounced enough that it would make you sit up and take notice.

Paresthesia would also make those of us in the ED rush you up to the radiology suite for testing, because it's the feeling you might get at the onset of a stroke.

"What's the algorithm?" my husband's friend asked.

"Well," the neurologist said, smirking. "When they come in, the first thing I ask is, 'Are they male or female?' If they're male, I say, 'Let's do a CT scan.' And if they're female, I say, 'Stop! It's anxiety. It's all in her head.'"

As my husband shared this story, I gaped at him, aghast. "You have got to be kidding me."

My husband shrugged uncomfortably. "It was just locker room talk. He wouldn't actually *do* that."

Locker room talk. Sure. We've all heard that one before.

When a prominent neurologist, well respected in his field and with what looks on paper to be a solid track record, makes statements like this—even supposedly in jest—it reveals the true depth of our medical community's prejudice against women. Rather than considering that a woman might be having an actual stroke, he would default immediately to a psychogenic diagnosis.

Healthcare professionals bring a lifetime of internalized beliefs, social constructs, and cognitive biases to work with them every day in addition to their wealth of actual clinical experience. These filters create expectations, preconceptions, and recognition tools; for example, we can often identify conditions without extensive testing because we've seen them before. However, these filters, when not examined, can also create biases that color providers' views of every-thing in their worlds—including the women they treat.

It isn't just male providers who carry these biases; depending on their social conditioning, women can be even less empathetic than men toward other women.

And yet, if you asked most healthcare providers, they would say that they aren't biased at all—that they are thoroughly objective and make their evaluations on a situation-by-situation basis. This is the nature of unconscious bias, and its immeasurability makes it even harder to eradicate.

In our society, women are often regarded as weaker than men, more prone to emotional outbursts, less able to tolerate discomfort and pain, and more likely to exaggerate their feelings in the hope of "getting attention." Despite the massive strides that women have made toward equality in the last sixty years, this perception persists.

What this means in real-time medical practice is that women's complaints are not believed. Like Lydia, they tell their providers over and over what they feel and sense in their bodies—only to be told that they're making it up.

It's true that it's more socially acceptable for women to show emotion than it is for men. But the act of showing emotion does not mean that a woman is "hysterical." It does not mean that she is exaggerating or making a play for sympathy or attention. It sim-ply means that she is communicating how she feels. However, be-cause men are more likely to be "stoic" (i.e., to repress or conceal their emotions), women in our society who show how they feel are deemed "weak" or unreliable, while men are seen as "strong and steady." When this perception is in play, providers and medical staff are statistically more likely to disregard what a woman says—whether or not they realize they are doing it.

One prominent manifestation of unconscious bias is the assumption that female symptoms are more likely to have an emotional cause. For example, in one study of patients with similar symptoms of irritable bowel syndrome (IBS), researchers found that men were more likely to be referred for X-rays, while women were offered antianxiety medication and lifestyle advice.[1] A retrospective study discovered that emergency providers were less likely to comply with Centers for Disease Control and Prevention guidelines for documentation and treatment of sexually transmitted infections when their patients were women, specifically with regard to complete documentation of symptoms and discharge instructions.[2] A 2012 study found that severely injured women were less likely to be brought to an ED or other trauma center by emergency medical service/paramedic personnel (49 percent of women versus 62 percent of men). Once other variants had been accounted for, study authors concluded that gender does play a role in victims' access to trauma care and that "the reasons for this differential in access might be related to perceived difference in injury severity, likelihood of benefiting from trauma center care, or subconscious gender bias."[3] And, as we learned in Chapter 3, women are less likely to be referred for appropriate cardiac testing and are often given inappropriate or ineffective diagnostic tests;[4] when these tests don't reveal classic male-pattern symptoms, a default diagnosis of anxiety is often applied.

It all comes back to the mistaken belief that women inherently exaggerate and amplify their symptoms. Yes, women are more likely to have an observable emotional response to whatever is happening in their bodies—but that does *not* negate what is happening physically.

In fact, as we'll explore in the next section, the female response to stress correlates in many ways to the symptoms of anxiety. But anxiety as a symptom and anxiety as a root cause are two drastically different things—and confusing the two can have life-threatening consequences for women.

Anxiety Should Be the Diagnosis of Exclusion, Not the Diagnosis of Default

Recently, I met Lindsey J. Gurin, MD, a neuropsychologist whose office is a repository for "lost cases." Whenever doctors in her network can't figure out what is wrong with their female patients, they send them to her—because if the doctors can't figure out what's wrong, they assume that whatever's happening with these women must be psychosomatic.

Dr. Gurin told me about a patient who had excruciating spinal pain that went away every time she took Valtrex for her oral herpes. Her doctors said it was psychosomatic, probably related to her anxiety. She insisted that she had herpes in her spinal fluid; to her, it was the only thing that made sense, fit all her symptoms, and explained why Valtrex was the only thing that affected her pain level. All she wanted was for someone to order a lumbar puncture to see what was really happening, get the treatment she needed, and stop the pain.

Dr. Gurin couldn't understand how this woman had ended up in her office with an anxiety diagnosis. After all, it's well known that herpes maintains a latent state in the nerves of the spinal cord, so this wasn't an out-of-left-field assertion. "A lumbar puncture sounded reasonable to me," she said, shrugging. "So I ordered one."

Turns out, the woman did have cerebrospinal herpes. And because one person finally listened to her, she received the treatment she needed.

This story has a happy ending, but so many others don't. If my colleague hadn't been willing to listen to her patient, the woman might still be living with excruciating pain.

We've covered in previous chapters how anxiety has become the "go-to" diagnosis for women—meaning, when providers aren't sure what's wrong, anxiety is their default explanation. As you now know, the symptoms of anxiety can indeed mimic the symptoms of major diseases, such as heart attack and stroke, as well as a plethora of other ailments. So why, when a woman comes into her local ED with a racing heart, chest pain, and labored breathing, is she more likely to be given a diagnosis of anxiety than a man in the same situation? Why is a woman who comes in with abdominal pain more likely to be sent home with antianxiety meds than an IBS protocol?

The answer, of course, is the presence of implicit bias and society's conditioning of women to discount their own inner wisdom and apologize for their feelings instead of trusting them.

I've seen so many women come into the ED with heart attack–like symptoms. As they wait to be seen (which often takes longer than it should, because the symptoms of female-pattern heart attack are not as pronounced as those for men, and therefore they aren't prioritized in triage), women often "talk themselves down." They try to rationalize the way they're feeling, in part because they don't want to be seen as hysterical.

Perhaps when a woman calls her husband to tell him that she's in the ED, he asks her, "Are you sure it's not your anxiety acting up?" She considers this as she waits to be seen by the doctors on duty. Then, when the intern or resident shows up to speak to her, she says, "My chest hurts, and I feel really shaky, but…it's probably just my anxiety acting up." For some reason, she feels like she needs to apologize for her symptoms, and so she reaches for the least offensive explanation. Her physician, noting that she had self-reported anxiety, will now be more likely to dismiss her symptoms than to investigate them.

Once a diagnosis of anxiety is on a woman's record, every subsequent visit to providers will be colored by that one line item. "Oh, you have anxiety listed here. So you probably don't need that X-ray for your IBS; your anxiety is probably causing a flare in your digestive tissues, but it's likely not a blockage or other serious emergency." Or, "Oh, I see you have anxiety. Did you know that that can cause chest pains?"

Or, in the case of the neurologist I mentioned, "You have anxiety listed here. You're probably not having a stroke."

A study on cardiac misdiagnoses published in the *New England Journal of Medicine*, which looked at more than 10,000 cardiac patients, noted that women under the age of fifty-five who went to the ED with chest pain or other significant heart attack symptoms were *seven times more likely to be sent home* than their male counterparts. This more than doubled their risk of death and drastically impacted their outcomes otherwise.[5]

I observed an example of this dynamic playing out in my own emergency department recently.

A lot of women experience something called supraventricular tachycardia (SVT). This is an abnormal heart rhythm that comes and goes. The heart will, without warning, suddenly start to race. The woman will get short of breath and start to sweat. But the abnormal rhythm can come and go without warning—and, often, by the time she gets to the ED and is seen, her heart rate is back to normal.

Sandee was one of those women. She kept coming in with self-reported symptoms of a racing heart, flushing, and chest discomfort. She also had an anxiety diagnosis on her chart. And so, over and over, she was told, "You're having panic attacks."

"I know what a panic attack feels like," she replied. "This isn't the same."

Finally, she was sent home with a Holter monitor—basically a personal electrocardiogram (EKG) machine that monitors heart rate activity for twenty-four or more straight hours. When she came back, Sandee's results clearly showed that she was suffering from episodes of SVT. But if she hadn't insisted that something was happening beyond anxiety symptoms, she might not have gotten the treatment she needed to get her tachycardia under control.

I'm not the only educator working in my ED, and I can't be present for every patient interaction, but I still feel partly responsible when mistakes like this happen. Since we are a teaching hospital, it's my job to supervise the interns and residents and help them learn on the job.

"What do you think the solution to this situation would be?" I later asked my resident, who'd been the one to send her home originally.

Of course, she knew where I was coming from with this, but I was still pleased with her answer: "I think we should offer Holter monitors to women who exhibit classic SVT symptoms *before* we diagnose them with panic attacks."

In other words, instead of making anxiety the default diagnosis for women with a certain set of symptoms, we should consider it only *after* other physical factors have been ruled out.

The thing that really gets under my skin about all of this is that—at least in my ED—*a large percentage of the women who come in with a diagnosis of anxiety on their charts don't actually meet the diagnostic requirements for anxiety!*

Generalized anxiety disorder (GAD) and panic disorder (PD) are among the most commonly-diagnosed mental disorders worldwide. In the U.K., women are twice as likely to report symptoms of anxiety as men, and nearly 25% of women over the age of 16 have reported some form of mental health challenge. However, both GAD and PD have specific symptoms. However, both disorders have specific symptoms associated with them. The *Diagnostic and Statistical Manual for Mental Disorders* (known as the *DSM*) defines GAD as

A) Excessive anxiety and worry (apprehensive expectation), occurring more days than not for at least six months, about a number of events or activities (such as work or school performance).

B) The individual finds it difficult to control the worry.

C) The anxiety and worry are associated with three (or more) of the following six symptoms (with at least some symptoms having been present for more days than not for the past six months): Restlessness, being easily fatigued, difficulty concentrating (or mind going blank), irritability, muscle tension, sleep disturbance.

D) The anxiety, worry, or physical symptoms cause clinically significant distress or impairment in social, occupational, or other important areas of functioning.

E) The disturbance is not attributable to the physiological effects of a substance (e.g., a drug of abuse, a medication) or another medical condition (e.g., hyperthyroidism).

F) The disturbance is not better explained by another medical disorder.

The American Psychiatric Association, which produces the *DSM*, is clear that "feeling anxious sometimes" or anxiety about one symptom or event does not constitute GAD. These guidelines also clearly state that other common physical and mental issues should be conclusively ruled out before a diagnosis of GAD is applied.

In my experience, a large percentage of women who are given a diagnosis of anxiety do not actually meet the *DSM* criteria for this specific (and truly debilitating) condition. But seeing this diagnosis in your medical chart invites a huge set of assumptions about everything from physical symptoms to emotional responses and can drastically color your doctor's impression of your subjective retelling of your symptoms. It will impact which tests are ordered, which medications are prescribed, and whether certain physical symptoms are dismissed as "normal" or treated as warning signs of something more serious. In short, this one offhand note in your chart about your anxiety could lead to a plethora of misdiagnoses—up to and including mistaking a heart attack for a panic attack.

Of course, there are many women out there who legitimately struggle with GAD (and PD, its cousin) every single day. I am in no way attempting to minimize their experience here. In fact, women with full-blown GAD may be even *more* likely to be misdiagnosed because of the severity of their physical symptoms.

But what about the women who don't meet the clinical definition of GAD? Why do they keep getting handed these anxiety diagnoses? The answer may lie in how the female body deals with stress.

A study published in the *Industrial Psychiatry Journal* titled "Gender Differences in Stress Response: Role of Developmental and Biological Determinants" found that men and women had measurably different responses to acute stressors in laboratory settings, including "activities of the Hypothalamic-Pituitary-Adrenal (HPA) axis (eg, cortisol) and sympathetic nervous system (eg, heart rate and blood pressure)."[6]

The study determined that "HPA response patterns differ markedly between males and females." Without getting too technical, the study basically concluded that while men are more likely to exhibit the classic "fight or flight" response to stress, women are more likely to operate on a "tend and befriend" model, which increases limbic activation. (The limbic system is the part of the brain responsible for processing emotion and memory.) The study went on to say that "HPA hyperactivity is a common finding in major depression, social phobia, panic disorder, generalized anxiety, obsessive-compulsive disorder, susceptibility to infectious diseases, and cardiovascular disorders." So the same heightened stress response that characterizes GAD can also be present in cardiovascular disease—in a way that's completely unique to women.

While much more research is needed to bear out the findings of this and other studies, it's my personal feeling that, to those who don't know what to look for, the normal female response to stress can *look* like anxiety without actually *being* anxiety.

Of course, the flip side of this would be to say that all women are medically "anxious" when under stress—which is what I'm afraid is happening on a widespread basis with anxiety misdiagnoses. We are only seeing the tip of the iceberg in terms of the repercussions of this—but it makes studying men and women differently even more imperative.

While those of us who know the difference are working to change this literally life-threatening trend, it's vitally important for women to advocate for themselves (whether or not they believe that they truly suffer from anxiety).

You own the information in your medical record. You can ask for copies in order to have more collaborative discussions with your doctors. And if there are notes or diagnoses in there that you feel are inaccurate, you can request that they be changed. (Just note that you will probably be asked to provide reasoning and/or evidence for this change before a provider will consent to make it.)

But, if you do ask to review your medical record, I want to give you fair warning: you may be assigned yet another inaccurate and undesirable label....

The "Complainers"

There is a segment of women that many within the medical system call "the complainers." Basically, when some providers see a folder full of test results, specialist visits, and various diagnoses, the assumption isn't that the woman is being improperly diagnosed. The assumption is that she's making it up—that she's "one of the crazy ones."

I'll admit that a small segment of the patient population *can* be challenging. There are people whose worries about their symptoms far outweigh the actual risks. (Studies show that about 4 to 6 percent of patients who visit EDs and urgent care centers suffer from hypochondriasis, or "illness anxiety disorder," according to *DSM* criteria.)[7] There are also people who make up illnesses in order to get attention. And, of course, there are a few patients who seem to love arguing with their doctors for no discernable reason.

But the vast majority of the time, I find that the "complainers" are not exaggerating, or overblowing, or stirring up drama. They have legitimate concerns, and those concerns are—for myriad reasons—being minimized.

For example, a woman might see her general practitioner about her ongoing chest pain. When her stress tests don't reveal any (male-pattern) warning signs of heart disease, she may be told that it's probably acid reflux or gastroesophageal reflux disease (GERD). She may be sent to a gastroenterologist, who tells her it's not reflux, but maybe it's a muscle pull. She then goes to the orthopedist, who says everything is structurally fine, but maybe her anxiety is acting up. So she goes to her general practitioner, who prescribes antianxiety medication and suggests she see a counselor. In the meantime, she's accumulating a folder full of tests and data that offer no clue as to the actual problem.

She may start asking herself, What am I supposed to do? I know something's wrong, but no one can figure out what's happening! She may, understandably, actually start feeling anxious at this point as a result of her natural stress response, which compounds her symptoms. Perhaps she goes to her local ED for the fourth or fifth time, at which point the attending physician looks at her overflowing folder and says to himself, *Oh, boy. Here's a complainer,* and sends her home with a pain reliever and a suggestion to "take it easy for a few days"—not because he doesn't want to help but because everything he knows to do has already been done, to no avail.

After presenting to a group of female physicians recently, I spoke to Paula J. Rackoff, MD, a rheumatologist who recently had a "complainer" referred to her practice by a colleague. The patient had been experiencing back pain, side abdominal pain, neck pain, and general malaise on and off for years. She arrived in Dr. Rackoff's office with a notebook full of recorded symptoms. Her electronic medical record was overloaded with test results that were all negative or "inconclusive."

"She kept apologizing to me," Dr. Rackoff told me. "She kept saying, 'I'm not making this up! You have to believe me!' I ended up ordering a battery of tests, even though in the back of my mind, I was thinking, What will I tell her if there isn't anything there to find?"

Turns out, there *was* something to find. The patient had been suffering from Crohn's disease. Not only were her intestines badly damaged, but the inflammatory process had been affecting her whole body and causing all her symptoms.

"After making the diagnosis, I sent her to a gastroenterologist, and the patient got on the right meds," Dr. Rackoff said. "She's feeling better for the first time in years."

When "complainers" come into my ED, they stand out to me as people who need a little more of my time than the standard patient. Often, when I am able to spend this time, their stories come out—just as Lydia's did. They tell me how their symptoms are affecting so many aspects of their lives and how their providers don't believe them when they say, "Something is wrong with me!"

Knowing what I do about women's bodies and symptoms, I give them a fresh look. I order new tests and review the tests already in their files. Most of all, I try to get to what they really want out of our time together. Is it a diagnosis? Is it to feel better? Is it simply to be heard, even if I don't have all the answers for them right now? Often I end up referring these patients to specialists in my network who can offer tests that will clarify what is really happening and get them the treatment they need.

At the very least, I can reassure them that they aren't crazy and that it's not all in their head.

Taking It Home

Addressing implicit bias against women in medicine can feel like a daunting task. I see it in action every single day, and it makes me furious. However, I don't think that the solution is for women to storm into their providers' offices in a rage and demand to be treated fairly. Although it might be initially satisfying, unfortunately, that kind of approach only serves to reinforce the very unconscious biases we are working to unravel.

Anger is, however, potent fuel for advocacy and hugely constructive in that channel. Take your righteous anger into the spaces where funding, research, and high-level protocol decisions are being made. Support female doctors and scientists in your community and help them get their voices heard. (A research team from Stanford University's Gendered Innovations program recently found a link between female research study authors and gender-based analysis.[8] In other words, women think about women's issues!) Talk to your local research institutions and national disease foundations about funding studies that look at implicit bias and how it impacts women. Share what you've learned in this book on social media and with your networks.

And for goodness' sake, don't apologize for being in pain, or frustrated, or just flat out steaming mad!

On the other hand, when it comes to dealing with your providers and any unconscious biases that might be present there, the key isn't attrition but education. Behavioral science tells us that people are unlikely to change when confronted; education and reasonable discussion are much more likely to produce results. And let's face it: your healthcare providers are people, just like anyone else.

So, how can women educate their providers?

1. First, you can educate *yourself* about your health—both the disease issues you may be facing and your overall health as a woman. (What you're learning in this book is a great start; don't be afraid to bring it with you to your appointments! Especially useful will be the conversation starters you'll find in Part III.) Ask for copies of everything that's in your medical chart and review that information as best you can— especially if you have an unfounded anxiety diagnosis.

2. Make every effort to "clean up your side of the street," as they say. Be clear about your medical history. Keep an up-to-date list of your prescriptions with you at all times. Clearly communicate what's happening in your body right now. Don't hide, minimize, or apologize for anything in your medical history. Even before sex differences are accounted for, your providers need *all* the relevant information about your conditions to make informed diagnoses and recommendations. Remember, even though tests and procedures are a large part of our process, they're only useful if we have a good idea of what we're looking for.

3. Ask questions. *Lots* of them. Ask for detailed explanations of your medical conditions, prescriptions, and any side effects you may need to watch for. Feel free to say, "Can you explain this to me in nonmedical terms so I can understand it better?" Asking for clarification doesn't make you look stupid. It makes you an informed consumer of modern medicine. (If you need help formulating your questions, I'll give you some detailed pointers in Chapter 10.)

4. Have all the facts. If you tend to get nervous speaking to doctors (or even if you don't), having a list of all the relevant information at hand for each appointment can be

very helpful in directing the conversation. For example, you might write out the following:

- Your past medical history
- Your surgical history
- All current and past pharmaceuticals, including dosing
- Any over-the-counter medications you're taking, including pain relivers like Advil or Tylenol, vitamins, antacids, and so forth
- Any recent tests and/or imaging and their results, including X-rays, CT scans, ultrasounds, EKGs, MRIs, stress tests, and so forth
- Any allergies to foods, medications, and other substances

5. And, finally, if you truly do suffer from anxiety and have symptoms different from those you normally deal with, be sure to articulate to your provider exactly what is different about how you're feeling now versus how you feel during a panic attack or other anxiety-related episode. Again, it might be helpful to write out a description beforehand, when you're feeling calm. Putting words to even the smallest differences can make a huge impact when it comes to getting the treatment you need.

What Matters—Your Key Takeaways

- Women are overall more likely to be given a psychiatric diagnosis than a physical one for a wide range of conditions.
- Anxiety is the diagnosis of default for women, meaning that when certain symptoms are present but providers can't tell what's wrong, they often assume it must be anxiety related.

- Implicit bias makes it more difficult for women to get accurate diagnoses and treatment, particularly for diseases whose symptoms resemble those of anxiety.
- Women need to stop apologizing and deflecting in conversations with their providers. Instead, they should be clear about their symptoms and how they feel and trust their sense of what is happening in their own bodies.

chapter six

A DEEPER SENSITIVITY: THE FEMALE RELATIONSHIP TO PAIN

I WAS WORKING the overnight shift not long ago when a woman came in with vulvar pain.

Yes, vulvar pain. Her whole perineal area was so inflamed and swollen that she couldn't even sit down. And no one could figure out what might be causing it.

I got her on sign-out, which meant I was responsible for determining whether she could go home, even though the exams performed by the previous attending physician hadn't produced any answers for her.

I grabbed my resident, saying, "Let's go see her. We need to get into her head space and see if there's anything we can do."

I could see the moment I opened the curtain that she was in real distress. A few minutes into our conversations, I'd learned that the woman, whose name was Margaret, was seeing her primary care doctor about this issue and had an MRI scheduled for a few days later, but she couldn't wait until then to find a solution to her pain. The Tylenol she was taking at home wasn't even taking the edge off.

In a lilting Yorkshire accent, Margaret told me that this pain had been going on unabated for weeks, and she still didn't have any answers. She was hoping the upcoming MRI would provide them, but even that wasn't certain.

I wanted to be able to offer her some relief—to give her a reset point—so I offered morphine.

"No," she said. "It's awful, the way that makes me feel. It's worse than the pain."

"Has there been anything that actually worked for you?" I asked.

"The first time this came on, I came here in an ambulance, and they gave me something in an IV. I think it began with a *T*? That helped for a while. But nothing else has."

"I think you're talking about Toradol. That's one of the alternatives I was going to recommend. Let's get you set up with that."

Even though I wasn't able to offer Margaret more than a few hours of relief from her pain, she was incredibly grateful. As the Toradol took effect, her whole body began to relax. You could literally see the tension go out of her face and shoulders. By the time she called her sister to drive her home, she was yawning.

"This will be the first good night's sleep I've had in days," she said.

Margaret was well cared for by medical standards. Her primary care physician was doing everything she could to figure out the problem and even responded to our middle-of-the-night request for more information. But while the wheels were turning and tests had been scheduled, Margaret was still waiting in pain—and that pain was bad enough to drive her out of her house and into the ED at 2:00 a.m.

I see a lot of frustrated women come and go through the doors of my emergency department. They're between tests or doctor's visits, and for myriad reasons, they aren't getting the answers they need and deserve. They come in because they can't see any other way to get through the day or the night. They aren't "drug seeking"; like Margaret, they just want to be able to function until someone helps them figure out what's wrong.

Why Do We Minimize Women's Pain?

Pain is the primary reason that people of either sex seek medical care. Most of the time, a person who ends up in the ED is in pain—whether it's from an acute condition like heart attack or appendicitis, a trauma injury like a broken bone, or something not yet diagnosed like Margaret's vulvar pain. Pain is the way our bodies tell us that there's something wrong.

You might think that because it's present across the spectrum, pain would be treated equally regardless of sex or gender. But this is demonstrably untrue. In fact, the way people receive care for pain is sharply divided between the sexes.

Women are less likely to receive adequate treatment for their pain. They are less likely to receive pain medication in a timely manner and at an appropriate dose. And they are more likely than men to receive a psychiatric diagnosis when they report pain symptoms.[1] (Yes, the anxiety misdiagnosis rears its head again here.)

It's been demonstrated that women have both a lower pain tolerance and a lower pain threshold than men. They are more likely to have higher pain scores than men for the same conditions, are more likely than men to report both acute pain and chronic pain, and are more likely to seek treatment for their pain.

Such facts are often tossed around in medical circles to minimize women's pain—to write women off as overly sensitive or brand them as attention-seeking—but I have the opposite view. I think the flaw is in our knowledge, research, and protocols. The fact is, we don't fully understand the differences in how men and women experience pain—so expecting the genders to be equivalent is an exercise in faulty reasoning.

The only tools we have to evaluate pain are subjective. Yes, we can measure vital signs—like heart rate, breathing rate, and blood pressure—but these aren't reliable indicators of pain. They only get us in the ballpark. The rest of our pain evaluation protocols include pain scales ("On a scale of one to ten, your pain is…") and visual analog tools ("Pick the emoji that corresponds to your pain level"). These are communication tools but hardly useful for gathering objective data.

Even the research quoted to prove that women have a lesser pain tolerance than men was based on observing people of different sexes whose hands and arms were plunged into buckets of ice water or whose fingers were attached to electrical stimulation equipment.[2] Women described the pain as having reached "intolerable" levels before men did and therefore were determined to have a lower pain tolerance than men, who stayed with the sensation longer. However, does this behavior actually determine tolerance? Or do women simply have more sensitivity on multiple levels to sensation that might result in the loss of life or limb? Were women's brains making the connection that "this pain might damage me," evaluating the possibility of lasting repercussions, and retreating from the pain based on a series of connected mental and physical factors? Or were they simply less tolerant of the cold? It's impossible, at this juncture, to guess with any certainty, but these are interesting questions.

Furthermore, it's been my observation and experience—and this, too, is subjective—that women are, for the most part, simply more attuned to their own bodies than men are. This may be a function of our biological ability to bear children (and our need to sense their growth within us) or simply the way our nervous systems are wired. Whatever the reason, women are more likely to notice symptoms when they first appear and seek treatment more frequently and earlier than men—as if they are hearing their bodies whisper, "Something's not right." Men, on the other hand, seem to be more likely to ignore symptoms and/or resist seeking treatment, in part because of the persistent gender-based expectation that they will "act manly" and "suck it up." This is supported by sports literature around concussions; men will often refrain from telling their coaches about possible head injuries because they don't want to be taken out of the next play.

Unfortunately, I'm in the minority with my viewpoint on gender differences. In the eyes of far too many practitioners in my field, it's a clinical fact that women simply are more likely to report pain—aka, more likely to "complain"—than men; therefore, their pain is often treated as less serious. As you can imagine, this has significant consequences for women, particularly those with chronic pain or pain disorders.

I consider it a big part of my job to educate other medical providers about the sex and gender differences we *do* understand about pain and pain pathways and—since pain is such a huge factor in when, why, and how people seek medical treatment—to help them take these differences into account when serving their patients. It's our responsibility to be open to new data about the differences in pain responses, pathways, and treatments between the sexes and to change our approach accordingly—even if that means challenging our own long-held beliefs.

The Physiology of Pain and Pain Relief

The more I research this subject, the more I come to understand that women aren't just more "sensitive" to pain than men. They actually *process pain differently* than men—physiologically, biologically, and psychologically, from the cellular level up.

It seems obvious, therefore, that women's pain must be treated, managed, and even identified according to different criteria. However, because the majority of our current pain research is based on male models, this is not currently being done.

A major reason, of course, for these differences is our sex hormones. Most cells produce and respond to sex hormones (such as androgens, estrogens, and progestins)—including nerve cells in the central nervous system (CNS). More, sex hormones directly affect both the organization and function of the CNS, starting in the womb. This means that neurotransmission—including the perception of and response to pain—is biologically different in men and women.

The areas of the brain that control perception of pain and analgesia (pain reduction or suppression) have receptors for both estrogens and androgens. Estradiol, a variant of estrogen, seems to be particularly important in controlling the structural and molecular aspects of the CNS because it regulates proteins involved in signal transduction. Estrogen in the bloodstream also appears to affect other neurotransmitters like dopamine and serotonin. This is why, for example, migraines are more prevalent during certain points in the menstrual cycle; decreased estrogen levels lead to decreased receptivity to serotonin.

Sex hormones also bind to nerve receptors in the brain, the spine, and peripherally throughout the body. They help to modulate the perception of and response to pain and can even lead to the formation of additional receptors that control pain response.

When something happens to cause pain, nociceptors—the sensory nerves responsible for recognizing pain—are stimulated. It's the job of nociceptors to transmit a pain signal to the CNS, where a response is formulated. However, along the way, different factors may modify the signal (i.e., the sensation), either intensifying or alleviating it.

In essence, pain medications intercept or ameliorate in some way the signals sent from the nociceptors to the brain. But because pain reception and perception is so strongly affected by sex hormones, because of the unique nature of female inflammatory responses, and because of differences in the ways that female cells communicate pain to the central nervous system, women respond differently than men to many treatments.[3] In fact, what works in men is not guaranteed to work to the same degree—or at all—in women.

This was demonstrated in animal models by Robert E. Sorge, PhD, an assistant professor at the University of Alabama in Birmingham, and his colleagues. In male and female mice with persistent pain and inflammation, they injected one of three drugs that inhibit microglial function (the mediation of immune response in the central nervous system). All three drugs reversed pain sensitization in the male mice but had no effect whatsoever in the females.[4]

While it's understood in the medical community that results in animal models may not be replicated exactly in humans, the fact that this study showed an entirely different process between male and female mice was highly intriguing and demonstrated the need for similar studies in humans.

Another groundbreaking study, conducted in Texas, looked at patients with metastatic spinal tumors that were pressing on dorsal root ganglia (clusters of neurons in the dorsal roots of spinal nerves). Dorsal root ganglia are the main signaling centers for the central nervous system. In essence, they take information from various parts of the body and relay it to the brain. Researchers found that after the tumors were removed in these study patients, there were differences in male and female inflammatory responses to pain. In fact, they identified different *gene expressions* related to pain and inflammation in their male and female subjects. This means, in essence, that men's and women's bodies signal their brains differently when there is a problem. This led researchers to conclude that there are sex-based differences to neuropathic chronic pain responses.[5]

This is an intriguing concept to study, particularly in relationship to women's pain management. Unlike some other pain medications (like the microglial inhibitors studied by Dr. Sorge and his team), opiates *do* seem to work to manage women's pain—although women are more likely than men to experience unpleasant side effects from their use. This efficacy may explain why prescription rates for opiates like oxycodone (Percocet, OxyContin), hydrocodone (Vicodin), and many others are so much higher for women, particularly women of reproductive age. It may also partially explain why women are more likely than men to use opiates without a prescription to cope with chronic pain or to self-treat for emotional conditions like anxiety. Unfortunately, this prevalence can also create a pathway for addiction and misuse.

Like so much else in medicine, nearly all our pain protocols, medications, and treatment procedures are still based on male models, male animal experiments, and male-centric research. In fact, a recent review in the journal *Pain* noted that at least 79 percent of animal studies published in that journal over the last ten years included only male subjects, while 8 percent studied only female subjects, and 4 percent studied sex differences.[6] And yet, as we've observed, the results of these male-centric studies are then applied to women as if their biology were interchangeable with men's.

In order to give women more and better treatment options for their acute and chronic pain, we need to understand how their pain is sensed, transmitted, and managed internally—particularly when it comes to ongoing pain and chronic pain disorders. Because we don't understand women's specific pain pathways, we are essentially fire-hosing the problem, hoping that something will work. Imagine if we could develop medicine to target sex-specific pain signals and inflammatory patterns. Could we relieve women's pain with lower doses, fewer side effects, and fewer addiction issues?

Women have exponentially higher rates of pain disorders tied to neurological function, including fibromyalgia, lupus, and chronic fatigue syndrome. Could this be because of the ways in which our bodies process pain?

Men and women are both able to produce their own internal analgesics—compounds that help take the "edge" off the pain and reduce inflammation. This process is called diffuse noxious inhibitory control (DNIC). However, people with chronic pain or with pain disorders like fibromyalgia have lesser, or "blunted," DNIC activity. Also, mu receptors in the brain and spinal cord (which diminish pain sensation and are the receptors that opioids bind to) are more prevalent in men than in women and do not respond as robustly in women because they are dependent on estradiol levels, which fluctuate during the menstrual cycle. This may explain why both chronic pain and pain disorders are more common in women and respond less well to treatment.

There are drugs that appear to work for chronic pain in women, particularly neuropathic pain; for example, Neurontin (gabapentin) and Lyrica (pregabalin) are often prescribed for fibromyalgia, diabetic nerve pain, and other pain disorders. However, the exact mechanisms by which these drugs dampen nerve response in the female body are not well understood. (In fact, Neurontin is an antiseizure drug, not a pain reliever, and was not originally intended for use in nerve pain patients.) Because we don't fully understand female pain pathways, it often feels to me that we are throwing drugs at the problem to see what "sticks." This is obviously not ideal for patients—but it's not ideal for our medical system either, particularly because these drugs come with a laundry list of potentially serious side effects that often complicate an already problematic situation.

Another common practice is to prescribe antidepressants and/or antianxiety medication for chronic pain disorders. Increasing serotonin and dopamine levels does help make chronic pain more bearable—but, in the long run, it's not a cure. Until we understand more about the underlying causes and mechanisms of chronic pain conditions like fibromyalgia, offering relief is the best we can do.

The fact is, until we understand the physiology of female pain, we will not be able to treat it effectively, and we will keep coming up with "halfway there" solutions for the conditions that are dramatically affecting women's lives. Broadening our understanding will help us not only to finally give women the relief they're seeking from their acute and chronic pain but also to understand the differing mechanisms of drug metabolism, efficacy, and addiction between the sexes.[7]

It's Not Just PMS: Pain and the Menstrual Cycle

Because hormones play such a key role in pain reception and perception, women's pain—chronic or otherwise—is inextricably tied to the menstrual cycle. And where gender bias is present, this provides another excuse to minimize women's pain.

Most sex-differentiated pain conditions appear during or after puberty. As a girl's body matures, levels of estrogen and other sex hormones soar, and the menstrual cycle begins. These hormones act on a number of sites in both the central and peripheral nervous systems and in both reproductive and nonreproductive tissues. It is around this time that things like ischemic migraine headaches, irritable bowel syndrome, chronic constipation, chronic tension headache, and other issues come to light in their uniquely female expressions.[8]

Also, as we know, women have a greater prevalence of chronic pain disorders, migraine, and autoimmune diseases. Falling estrogen levels in the premenstrual period are associated with "flares" of these disorders. Areas of the brain that control perception of pain have receptors for estrogens, as well as for androgens like testosterone, dihydrotestosterone (DHT), and dihydroepiandosterone (DHEA). Estradiol, a form of estrogen, is particularly involved in signal transmission in the central nervous system. When its levels fluctuate, as they do naturally during a woman's menstrual cycle, susceptibility to and perception of pain can change as well. Therefore, when women at a certain point in their menstrual cycle have a "flare" of their pain disorder, their pain—the way their central nervous system perceives sensation—is *actually* increased. It's not a matter of perception. It's a matter of neural *reception*.[9]

The interactions of hormones with the CNS and neuroendocrine systems are well documented, as are the places in a woman's cycle where breakthrough episodes are common. However, when these women go to the ED or to their doctors, they're not likely to be asked questions like, "Where are you in your menstrual cycle?" Or "Have you noticed that you tend to get these migraines a week or so before your period?" Instead, they may be given medications or treatments that they may not need for the other three weeks out of the month. However, a provider who is aware of the link between menstrual cycles and pain may be *less* likely to offer treatment that will help during the few days of this flare; instead, women might receive that age-old brush-off: "It's just PMS. Wait a few days and you'll be fine."

To most people (including many women), PMS is just a part of life, something women have to live with. It's almost regarded as the price we pay for being women, a normal rite of passage that just happens to be worse for some women than for others.

It's true, PMS *is* a part of life as a biological female—but for some women, especially those with chronic pain disorders, it's an uncomfortable, even excruciating part. So why aren't we talking about it as a genuine, valid health complaint and seeking out ways to make it tolerable?

Not to sound glib, but if men had to undergo a cycle of testicular pain every month, you bet there would be validation, research, and new meds produced for them. Just like erectile dysfunction became "ED" and got its own sleek blue pill, men's monthly testicular pain would get an acronym (MTP!) and a designer pharmaceutical solution, along with support groups, television ads—the works. (Okay, maybe that's a bit over the top. But you can bet that monthly pain cycles wouldn't be something men "just had to live with.")

And yet pain flares associated with women's menstrual cycles are invalidated on a daily basis. Even if tests are performed to look for other potential causes for the pain, providers aren't always able to help women understand what's going on (likely because they aren't aware of the estradiol/pain link themselves), and so women's concerns are sidelined. Not only does this fail to help women in the moment, but if they feel like their doctors think they're exaggerating when they say, "It hurts," the likelihood that they will seek appropriate care in the future is significantly decreased.

While the link between estradiol and pain levels is understood, there are still many questions about how hormonal levels and fluctuations actually impact women's experience of pain. We know that it happens, but we aren't entirely certain *why*.

Two brain-imaging studies looked at whether differences in pain sensitivity in healthy women could be visually measured.[10] In one, painful heat was applied to the skin over the left masseter muscle (the muscle that connects the lower jaw to the cheekbone and facilitates the action of chewing). The pain response was measured at two points in women's cycles: once during a period of high estrogen and again during a period of low estrogen. While there was no significant difference in pain ratings between the two points, different activation patterns were observed in the brain. In another study, a finger was immersed in painfully hot water during low- and high-estrogen points in the subject's cycles. Here, as well, differences in brain activation were observed, but this time there were also differences in pain and "pain unpleasantness" ratings. This revealed that while hormone levels may or may not alter the neurotransmission aspect of certain kinds of pain, they do affect the person's perception and experience of pain—and that alteration is statistically measurable via brain scan.

What does this mean for women in pain? To me, it's evidence that we need to be looking at all this information a lot more closely. Whether it's a matter of reception, perception, or both, women's hormonal cycles can and do affect their experience of both acute and chronic pain. And as we learned in Chapter 4, hormone levels also affect the efficacy of pharmaceuticals, including pain relievers. Therefore, women's unique and fluctuating hormonal states should be taken into account whenever pain diagnoses and treatments are relevant.

Of course, this discussion of hormone levels must also affect peri- and postmenopausal women. As we know, falling estrogen levels create elevated pain states and pain perceptions; therefore, we can assume that permanent changes in hormone levels and cycles will also create changes in pain states and pain perception. (We'll explore this further in Chapter 7.) More study is needed to understand how menopause affects women's pain and pain sensitivity, but given what we now know, we should take this into account when treating older women.

Once we understand more completely how the menstrual cycle affects the central nervous system and pain perception in a holistic way, we will be able to more effectively treat pain based on where a woman is in her cycle and stage of life. Until then, we need to keep learning—but also keep listening, regardless of whether a woman's experience of pain agrees with our preconceptions.

"Yentl Syndrome": Turning Up the Volume

Recently, I saw a woman named Jennifer in the emergency department. It was her first visit to my hospital but her fourth visit to an ED in a week. She was experiencing intense abdominal pain on her right side and some vaginal bleeding and was incredibly distraught.

"People keep telling me that I probably just had an ovarian cyst that ruptured. But no one has actually done anything for me! They said my ultrasound showed 'free fluid in the pelvis' and that it would go away on its own, but I'm still in pain. And it seems like when I explained to the other doctors that I needed help, that the pain was getting worse, they just passed me off to someone else or tried to send me home!"

As she sobbed out her story, I could feel Jennifer's fear. And inside, I was cringing. *Just* a ruptured cyst? Ovarian cysts are common and do sometimes rupture. This isn't considered a medical emergency; while it is definitely painful, a rupture isn't usually dangerous and rarely requires surgery or additional treatment. However, if the cyst is large or complex, a rupture might cause internal bleeding, infection, and even death. Large cysts can also cause something called ovarian torsion, where blood flow is cut off to the ovary, causing severe pain and, if left untreated, cell death and irreparable damage to the ovary.

Obviously, the initial ultrasound Jennifer received had led her providers to believe that there was no need for additional intervention. But the pain and fear Jennifer was experiencing had already caused her to lose multiple days of work and life. And if the pain was getting worse instead of better, something else might be at play.

What caught my attention was the word "probably." A "probably" is a *guess*, not a diagnosis—even if, in this case, it was an educated guess based on an ultrasound—and uncertainty always sets my emergency physician mind to turning. Jennifer might have had a ruptured ovarian cyst, which would absolutely result in free fluid in the pelvis—but her escalating pain might be coming from something else entirely, like an ectopic pregnancy, pelvic inflammatory disorder, or even appendicitis.

"I'm so sorry you haven't gotten a diagnosis," I told her. "And honestly, the ED isn't always the best place to get one. We're not set up for extensive testing. I think you should call your OB/GYN for an appointment as soon as possible—but in the meantime, I'm going to recommend a CT scan to rule out other causes of severe abdominal pain, and we'll go from there."

The CT scan showed that Jennifer did, in fact, have fluid in her pelvic area consistent with a burst cyst. Luckily, there didn't appear to be any internal bleeding—so, in that regard, the initial diagnosis had been correct, and no additional treatment was necessary. However, she *did* have two other large cysts present that hadn't been revealed by the ultrasound; these could be contributing to the abdominal pain she was experiencing. I referred her to a surgeon so that she could discuss the risks and benefits of having them removed before they ruptured on their own.

Even though I wasn't able to send her home with a "cure"—the blood and fluid from her ruptured cyst would be absorbed by her body over the next several weeks—I was able to offer her some relief from her pain and a concrete explanation of what was happening in her body. In fact, I felt like the biggest part of my contribution wasn't just affirming the original diagnosis but witnessing Jennifer in her personal crisis. If she had to come to me after seeing so many other providers, just so I could tell her essentially the same thing, she didn't feel cared for or validated.

Jennifer's experience reinforced for me not only that female pain is treated differently but that how women *communicate* their pain is a huge factor in how that pain is treated. As Jennifer shared, the more she tried to explain her pain to her previous providers, the more they seemed to tune her out.

Unfortunately, this kind of thing happens all the time. It's a phenomenon called "amplification," and it's a gender-based perception bias that rears its head in hospitals and physician's offices around the country and the world.

I wrote about this in the paper I coauthored with my colleague Bruce Becker, MD, titled "Men, Women, and Pain."[11]

Inadequate treatment of a patient's pain during an acute episode of illness or injury will create a negative expectation on the part of that person, which will accompany that person to his or her next acute medical encounter, influencing that patient's approach to communicating the nature, quality, and intensity of the pain. It is likely that there will be an amplification effect. As the patient speaks louder about the pain (gives the pain more voice, metaphorically speaking), the healthcare provider may reflexively "turn down the volume" on their receptors, becoming less and less able to hear the patient's expressions of pain. The interpretation of this voice of pain rising in tone and timber will increasingly be tempered by the belief that the patient is exaggerating (which in a sense he or she is doing). Other important pieces of the medical conversation might then also be misconstrued, leading to delayed or inadequate diagnosis, mistreatment, and increased morbidity and mortality for the patient....Undertreatment of a patient's pain causes patient dissatisfaction, patient distrust, a form of PTSD [posttraumatic stress disorder], and anxiety associated with the medical visit. Thus a vicious cycling and amplification of behavior is engendered that is self-defeating for the patient and significantly undermines the provider-patient relationship. The behavior, once initiated, leads to misdiagnosis and mistreatment that is damaging to the patient and costly to the healthcare system.

In essence, the more a patient's pain is ignored, the more she will "amplify" her sharing of the pain in order to get the attention of those who can help. However, I know from experience that, in a busy ED, it's all too easy for doctors and nurses to tune out or minimize these cries for help. After all, we deal with patients in pain all day and night; sometimes, at the end of a long day, it's tempting to just push it all into the background and get on with the tasks at hand. This approach is not only lacking in compassion but dangerous for patients. And, as mentioned above, it creates a cycle of misdiagnosis, minimization, and additional pain for the patient—and, in the end, an increased burden on providers.

Amplification can happen whenever a patient in distress is not being heard. Many people, including physicians, have internalized a cultural perception of women as weaker, less tolerant of pain, and more prone to exaggerate and "blow things out of proportion." And because it's obvious to female patients when their doctors aren't responding to their distress, they *do* place more emphasis on their pain, because they're not being seen or heard. It's a truly vicious cycle.

In the medical world, this situation is dubbed the "Yentl syndrome." The term was coined by Bernadine Healy, MD, in 2001 to sum up the paradox of adverse outcomes experienced by women with ischemic stroke, as well as the prevalent underdiagnosis and undertreatment of women across the board. In essence, it describes any situation where a woman needs to prove to her providers that she is as sick as the men around her.[12]

I couldn't help but feel that this was exactly what had happened to Jennifer. Her complaint was minimized by the first person she encountered, and as her upset grew, her providers responded not with follow-through but by "turning down the volume" on everything she was saying. And because many providers are still not educated in the dynamics of pain communication, especially across genders, this cycle continued across three ED visits and multiple days.

Luckily, Jennifer's condition didn't merit emergency surgery. But the fact that her life wasn't in imminent danger didn't mitigate the trauma of having her fear, pain, and anxiety minimized. Her ruptured cyst wasn't considered an "emergency" by her providers (when compared to other possible diagnoses), but it was a crisis to her. Her negative experience will likely now color every interaction she has with her providers.

For other women, the amplification effect is devastating not only psychologically but physically. In a 2015 article in *The Atlantic*, Joe Fassler detailed the experience of his wife, Rachel, who suffered from ovarian torsion.[13] Her providers wrote her off as having kidney stones after asking only a few questions and without even a basic examination. The result was that she waited more than three hours for pain relief of any kind and more than fourteen hours for surgery. She ended up losing her ovary and suffering from trauma-related PTSD symptoms because no one—not her nurses, not her doctor—believed her pain levels were actually consistent with her expression of them.

Sex is not the only subjective element in pain diagnosis and management. There is still a pervasive, if largely subconscious, belief within the medical field that minorities, particularly black women, don't feel pain the same way that white people do. Therefore, the amplification effect may be exaggerated in situations where women of color are being vocal about their pain. We'll discuss this more in Chapter 8—but for now it's vital to understand that when women of color say they aren't being heard in medical situations, they're absolutely right.

There are also biases against cultural displays of pain. The term "status Hispanicus" is thrown around in some EDs because some Hispanic women have a cultural display of pain that is viewed as extreme. Women may physically rock back and forth, ululate, and otherwise vocalize their pain. For providers who don't understand this, it can seem like the woman thinks the world is ending over a broken toe—and so, a cycle of judgment and minimizing ensues.

There are layers upon layers of overt and subtle perceptions that affect the way physicians treat their patients, and, unfortunately, many of them end with women's pain being minimized—not necessarily in a clinical sense (although that can and does happen) but in the interactions with the individual. This isn't the case of a few "bad apples" or negligent providers; rather, it is a symptom of a system that has habitually excluded women in its research, clinical trials, and treatment models. We don't understand how to assess, treat, and simply be with women in their pain because we've never learned, as a collective, how to do so.

As a system, we understand even less how to treat and connect with women of color. If you are a woman of color, I encourage you to get even more specific in your observation of how stereotypes and assumptions may be affecting your quality of care on both micro and macro levels. As I've shared previously, education is always the solution when it comes to implicit bias—but until that education is widespread within the medical community, I encourage you to seek out facilities and providers where you are comfortable and feel seen and heard by both doctors and staff. Take note of any and all experiences where you feel bias is at play and speak out whenever and wherever you can.

Taking It Home

Treating pain is one of the most common and necessary things we do as physicians. But not all providers are educated about how to engage with women's pain. Therefore, it's up to us as women to ask the right questions, find the right solutions, and ensure that our concerns are heard.

First—and I know I've said this before, but I can't stress it enough—if you don't understand what's happening, don't be afraid to ask questions. It's okay to say that you are confused or that you don't understand the medical terminology being used. If you have pain but don't understand the diagnosis or feel as though your concerns are being minimized, ask your doctor to explain what's happening in a way you can understand and can repeat back to him or her in your own words. Or ask something like, "Can you write all this down for me so I can read it when I'm home and in a better space to understand what my next steps are?"

Second, understand what medications you are taking for your pain and why. Ask your primary care provider for a list of alternatives to opiates and other potentially addictive medications, and ask whether these have been tested in women. If you don't feel like your current medications are providing the relief you need, ask if there are others that might act on different sets of receptors and therefore be more effective in your female body.

Third, research alternative options for treating your pain. Acupuncture, in particular, has been shown in clinical trials to work on the same neuroreceptors (mu receptors) as opiates.[14] Other options like yoga, meditation, massage, and even Reiki can be useful adjunct therapies for both acute and chronic pain. Because hormone levels are affected by stress, finding ways to relax can make chronic pain more bearable.

Finally, when you are in pain, it's hard to be rational and cool-headed. Therefore, it's helpful to gain as much knowledge about your body and its response to pain as possible, even if you don't have a chronic pain issue and aren't likely to seek care for pain in the near future. This will help you to ask the right questions of your providers and make better decisions about your care in a potentially stressful situation.

What Matters—Your Key Takeaways

- Women have a biologically different pain mechanism and response than men—and these differences are only now coming to light.

- Women's hormonal cycles can and do affect pain levels, pain perception, and the efficacy of pain treatments. You are more likely to experience greater pain when your estrogen levels are low.

- Not all pain medications work as well for women as they do for men. If you feel like you're not getting the appropriate or expected level of pain relief from your medication, it may help to switch prescriptions, so talk to your provider.

- Women's expressions of pain are often subject to implicit bias on the part of providers, resulting in the "amplification effect." This is particularly true for women of color or whose cultural displays of pain are more vocal or demonstrative.

- Complementary therapies have been demonstrated to work as well as prescription drugs on certain types of pain in women and should be considered viable treatment options for women with chronic pain and pain disorders.

chapter seven

BEYOND HORMONAL: FEMALE BIOCHEMISTRY AND HORMONE THERAPY

I WAS WORKING an overnight shift when a young woman named Katie came into the ED. She was thirty years old and appeared to be in good health but was experiencing increased heart rate and pain in her upper chest when she took a deep breath, so we admitted her for some testing.

I looked over her paperwork: no apparent risk factors for cardiovascular disease; no previous hospital stays or surgeries; no prescriptions other than birth control pills.

"This sounds like pleuritic chest pain. Has this ever happened before?" I asked.

"Not like this," Katie replied, her voice shaking. "I sometimes get panic attacks, but this feels different."

There it was: the easy out. Anxiety, the go-to diagnosis in women. But this was something different.

"Katie, do you smoke?" I asked. "Like, when you're out drinking with friends? Or do you have a few cigarettes a day?"

"Um…sometimes? Yes. Both of those."

Katie hadn't indicated that she was a smoker on her intake questionnaire. This is common. Many women who are "social smokers" don't consider it a habit and don't understand the damage even those few weekly cigarettes can do.

"Katie," I said, "I'd like to check out a few things, including your heart and lungs. I want to rule out any possibility that you might have a blood clot."

Each year, upward of 100,000 people die of pulmonary embolism or deep vein thrombosis (DVT), both of which are forms of blood clots.[1] Women on hormonal birth control are, on average, at about four times higher risk of experiencing a blood clot than women who don't use hormonal contraceptives—but in context, this risk is still relatively small (under 1 percent for young, otherwise healthy women, about the same as for pregnant women).[2] However, when you add in cigarettes, things get really serious, because nicotine accelerates the heart rate and narrows the diameter of the blood vessels, making it easier for clots to form. Smoking also makes platelets "sticky," which encourages clotting.[3]

In all my years in the ED, I can't recall seeing an otherwise healthy thirty-year-old man with a blood clot in his lungs (unless he had a severe extenuating risk factor, like traveling by airplane on extended nonstop flights)—but Katie (who did, in fact, have a blood clot in her lung and needed immediate treatment) and many other women in her age group who use birth control come to the ED with clotting conditions every year. In fact, being on hormone-based birth control is an independent risk factor for clotting conditions. And while women are often warned of the dangers of smoking while on birth control, they aren't aware of how the hormones they're taking on a daily basis are affecting everything about their physiology and why such pharmaceuticals make conditions like Katie's blood clot more likely and more devastating for them across the board.

The New Female Biology

As we've learned in previous chapters, female hormones are not merely "disruptors" that influence mood and monthly menstruation. Women's hormones affect everything about their physiology, from their immunity to their circulatory systems to their response to pain and pain medications. Estrogens, progestins, and other female hormones affect cell function throughout the body; just as every cell in a woman's body contains female chromosomes, every cell has receptors for steroidal hormones. Estrogen, in particular, competes for vital "transporters" that bring it into the cell. These same transporters are also used by other chemical compounds, including some prescription drugs. This creates a complex dynamic wherein there is competition for the cells' "attention," which in turn affects what they ingest and how; the result is health patterns, concerns, and diseases that are mostly, or even exclusively, female.

When we add synthetic hormones to the mix, as Katie was doing with her birth control, women's unique risk factors can be altered or compounded. Many women use exogenous (meaning, manufactured or introduced from outside the body) hormones every day in a multitude of ways. The most ubiquitous of these uses, of course, is birth control—in forms ranging from oral contraceptives to hormone-excreting intrauterine devices (IUDs) to other implanted and transdermal contraceptive devices—but synthetic hormones are also prescribed after reproductive surgeries like hysterectomy and ovary removal, as well as to treat menopausal and perimenopausal symptoms, skin conditions, and even depression. We aren't always sure of the exact mechanisms that make these treatments effective (for example, the link between birth control pills and reduced acne is only partly understood); we simply know that many women find them helpful and often lifesaving.

Exogenous hormones are truly a gift for many women. They can bring the body into balance after surgery or menopause. They can relieve painful symptoms associated with premenstrual syndrome (PMS) and menopause. They can positively increase the effects of other important medications. And they can help women achieve a greater overall sense of well-being by improving sleep, mood, and vaginal dryness, allowing them to enjoy sex and intimacy more fully later in life.

However, exogenous hormones also come with a laundry list of side effects, many of which are "accelerations" or amplifications of phenomena we've already observed as part of women's unique biology. Katie's clotting issues were one example. Others include mood swings, weight gain, swelling, "brain fog," and increased risk of certain cancers.

Also, while some applications of exogenous hormones (such as birth control) have been well studied, others don't always work the way we expect them to. For years, physicians prescribed high-dose hormone replacement therapy (HRT) for postmenopausal women, thinking that it would reduce their risk of heart attack and stroke. After all, we'd observed the "estrogen protective effect" in younger women, and so it was natural to assume that this effect would translate to older women's bodies; observations noted in several research studies appeared to confirm this. However, the result was exactly the opposite of what was intended; use of high-dose exogenous hormones actually *increased* women's chances of blood clots, deep vein thrombosis, gallbladder disease, urinary incontinence, and stroke—all while producing no measurable effect on heart disease.

The landmark study that finally put the brakes on the unquestioned use of HRT for menopausal symptoms and heart attack prevention was the Women's Health Initiative, which looked at both estrogen-only therapy and estrogen-progestin therapy in postmenopausal women. The panel was looking at the effects of HRT on a number of chronic conditions, including heart disease. However, while findings did indicate that HRT could protect women from bone loss and hip fracture, it also revealed that neither therapy actually reduced cardiovascular risks. In fact, HRT produced an increase in susceptibility to the side effects mentioned above. The estrogen-plus-progestin group also showed an increased risk of pulmonary embolism, dementia, and invasive breast cancer.

In 2002, when it became clear that the risks—particularly around breast cancer—were statistically too severe to ignore, the trial was cut short. In just a few years, prescriptions for HRT in the United States dropped from 90 million to about 30 million.[4] Media coverage of the trial and its cessation fed into women's fears that the HRT they'd been promised would help them was actually killing them. In the U.K., the landmark Million Women study, which began in 1996, also found that HRT correlated with an increasing risk of breast and ovarian cancers; the resulting drop in HRT usage was similar to that in the U.S.

Now we have a much better understanding of how exogenous hormones work in the female body and in which dosages we should be prescribing them. (In all cases, the lowest effective dose is best.) We have also developed guidelines for the safe and effective use of HRT for women in different age groups. For example, research has found that estrogen therapy is generally safe for women of reproductive age, as well as during and up to ten years following menopause. It's also worth noting that no other therapies have been found to be as effective for alleviating symptoms like vaginal dryness, hot flashes, night sweats, and other common issues. However, ten years or more after menopause, the estrogen receptors on a woman's cells have actually atrophied due to disuse, and her body has created other hormonal communication pathways to transport vital chemicals and information. At this point, the introduction of exogenous estrogen can trigger an inflammatory response, putting the woman at greater risk of side effects, cancer, and cardiovascular events.

While HRT is nowhere near as risky as it was twenty years ago, it can still amplify certain risk factors for the women who are taking it, especially if they smoke, drink, are obese, or have other preexisting conditions. And if women are no longer being promised that HRT will grant them immunity from heart attacks, they *are* being prescribed HRT in various iterations for other common conditions, including depression, chronic pain syndromes, and the prevention of osteoporosis. This creates even more complexity, because these exogenous hormones are interacting not only with the woman's body but also with other pharmaceuticals.

The application of exogenous hormones for the treatment of chronic pain syndromes is a good example of this. As I shared in Chapter 5, we are now discovering that women's pain pathways are different from men's and that hormone levels impact pain perception and tolerance levels. We also know that dropping estrogen levels in the luteal phase of menstruation are associated with an increase in pain. Therefore, it seems natural to assume that introducing exogenous hormones would "level the field" in women's bodies and help to solve some important pain issues. However, a study conducted in 2001 observed that healthy older women who were using exogeneous hormones as part of an HRT regimen demonstrated *lower* pain thresholds and pain tolerances than their non-HRT counterparts.[5]

As you can imagine, this has far-reaching implications for women dealing with conditions like fibromyalgia and chronic fatigue syndrome. HRT is widely prescribed for such conditions, but the reality is that while monthly dips in hormone levels do seem to create pain flares, supplementing with synthetic hormones—in particular, estradiol—does not appear to reduce pain at all. A double-blind, randomized, placebo-controlled trial conducted in Sweden in 2010 by Anders Blomqvist, MD, et al., tellingly titled "Hormonal Replacement Therapy Does Not Affect Self-Estimated Pain or Experimental Pain Responses in Post-Menopausal Women Suffering from Fibromyalgia," found that while "sex hormones, and in particular oestrogens, have been shown to affect pain processing and pain sensitivity, and oestrogen deficit has been considered a potentially promoting factor for [fibromyalgia]…no differences in self-estimated pain were seen between treatment and placebo groups."[6] The authors concluded, "Eight weeks of transdermal oestradiol treatment [did] not influence perceived pain, pain thresholds or pain tolerance as compared with placebo treatment in post-menopausal women suffering from [fibromyalgia]."

To me, this is an indication of two things. First, we don't fully understand the relationship between female hormones and female-pattern disease. And second, exogenous hormones may not operate in exactly the same way within the body as endogenous hormones—those produced by the body. Therefore, we need to study the mechanisms of these therapies more deeply in order to understand when and how to use them effectively. In cases like those described above, the risks of HRT may outweigh the benefits.

One place where HRT appears to be helpful is in the treatment of depression. A Chinese study looked at the alleviation of depressive symptoms associated with menopause. Participants were divided into two groups. One was given cyclic estrogen/progesterone, and the other was given both the HRT and a standard dose of fluoxetine (an antidepressant sold under the brand name Prozac). Participants in the second group saw a 92 percent "healing" rate, while HRT alone produced a 48 percent healing rate.[7] I found this interesting, because it demonstrated the relationship between female hormones and the ways in which drugs are assimilated in the body.

Another study published in the *Journal of Affective Disorders* correlated these findings, demonstrating that HRT increased the effects of selective serotonin reuptake inhibitors (SSRIs) in patients with major depressive disorders.[8] There also appear to be cases in which taking SSRIs decreased the prevalence of symptoms typically associated with menopausal hormone disruption, such as hot flashes or mood swings.

In my own experience, it's not uncommon for both pre- and postmenopausal women to be prescribed hormones for a multitude of symptoms. Many younger women find relief from PMS symptoms, skin conditions, and painful periods by taking oral birth control pills, regardless of whether they are sexually active. Literally hundreds of clinical studies have proven the effectiveness of HRT for lessening or preventing menopausal symptoms, bone loss, and mood swings. And women of all ages are prescribed exogenous hormones to potentiate the effects of other medications or to alleviate symptoms of various conditions, as we see with fibromyalgia.

However, as with all pharmaceuticals, we need to weigh the risks and benefits of prescribing hormones for any reason, including for birth control. More, we need to be precise and clear about communicating the potential risks of exogenous hormones to women who need or choose to take them. Perhaps, had the potential implications of her few weekly cigarettes been communicated more clearly to Katie, she could have avoided a potentially life-threatening clot in her lungs.

Above all, we need to acknowledge what we don't yet know. Since we don't understand all the mechanisms of exogenous hormones in the body, we don't know how they will impact, potentiate, or negate many other important pharmaceuticals. This gap in knowledge should be made clear to women who choose to undertake a hormone regimen—but it also shouldn't be a blanket deterrent. Many women benefit greatly from hormone therapy and experience increased quality of life in multiple areas as a result.

A Dual Biology: Exogeneous Hormones and Transgender Persons

It's clear that we have only scratched the surface of how exogenous hormones affect and interact with both our bodies and other pharmaceuticals. But an even bigger gap in our knowledge about how exogenous hormones affect health impacts the most misunderstood and marginalized individuals of all: transgender men and women.

Most medical practitioners don't understand the unique physiological needs of this population, especially when someone is actively "in transition." Some relegate the desire to transition to a different biological sex to a simple gender identity issue; others dismiss or ignore it on religious grounds. However, regardless of anyone's personal standpoint on the situation, the fact is that gender transition creates an overlap between someone's birth sex (and the presence of the associated hormones, pain pathways, XX or XY chromosomes, etc.) and new sex (with its different balance of hormones, which affect so many basic physiological processes). And because hormones are at play in so many daily bodily functions, we need to understand how exogenous hormones affect not just cisgender (matching biological sex and gender) female bodies but also the bodies of those in transition.

Questions abound. For example, should we prescribe medication based on biological sex as assigned at birth or on the reassigned sex and the hormones being used to aid/sustain the transition? If a person no longer has a penis and testes and is taking estrogen and antiandrogens to transition, should we still prescribe general medications based on the male chromosome model (XY) and according to male dosing? After all, this transgender woman still has XY-chromosomal cells in her liver and kidneys, which are processing and excreting the medicine; how is the estrogen affecting those?

This is a giant gray area, and the research hasn't come close to catching up to the daily reality. In fact, many providers fail to ask simple questions like, "Which organs do you have?" or "How far along in your transition are you?" Or even "Which types and doses of hormones are you taking?"

Much more study is needed before we can fully understand the holistic effects of exogenous hormones for gender transition. However, what we *do* know—and what I find extremely compelling—is that taking exogenous hormones puts people at risk for many of the disease patterns of their *new* sex in addition to those of their former or birth sex.

Transgender women (individuals born with male sex characteristics who are transitioning/have transitioned to female bodies) are more likely to experience female-pattern coronary disease.[9] Many trans women take the drug spironolactone (which suppresses androgens like testosterone) as well as "female" hormones like estrogen. The result is an increased risk of deep vein thrombosis, pulmonary embolism, and blood-clotting disorders; these factors are similar, in fact, to the risks of cis women like Katie who are taking oral contraceptives. Therefore, individuals who have clotting disorders, smoke, are obese, or have other risk factors for coronary or microvascular diseases should weigh the benefits of such prescriptions for gender transition against the potential side effects and speak with their providers about how to be sure they're taking the lowest effective dose of the necessary hormones. Trans women are also at increased risk for both asystole (flatlining) and torsades de pointes (see Chapter 4) and appear to have a decreased incidence of male-pattern heart issues like ventricular fibrillation.

This raises the question, *Is it our chromosomes or our hormones that underpin and influence our disease patterns?*

On the flip side, transgender men (individuals born with female sex characteristics who are transitioning/have transitioned to male bodies) are at increased risk for male-pattern diseases when they start taking exogenous testosterone. Potential complications include high blood pressure, elevated cholesterol, and diabetes, as well as mental and emotional side effects like aggression and neurotic behaviors. While these potential side effects may not adversely affect someone who is young and healthy, if you're someone who already suffers from hypertension, high cholesterol, elevated triglycerides, or circulatory issues, it's important to understand what adding testosterone to the mix might precipitate.

Studies have also found that trans men undergo several changes to mood and brain function as a result of taking exogenous testosterone. Brain scans have found increased connectivity between the temporoparietal junction (involved in own-body perception) and other brain areas, which has the effect of increasing the "fight or flight" response.[10] Mood changes, such as increased aggression and neurotic behaviors, have also been observed. Overall brain volume also increased with testosterone use—particularly in the hypothalamus, which (among other tasks) monitors hormone secretions.[11] Therefore, individuals who suffer from compulsive disorders, anxiety, previous hormonal imbalances, and mood disorders should be cautious when introducing testosterone; it may be necessary to increase or adjust existing mediations to ameliorate the effects of the hormone therapy.

For me and for other physicians who work with transgender individuals, risks like these merit a high level of attention. While studies are starting to emerge about the effects of hormones for gender affirmation on transgender persons' brains and bodies, whenever you start adapting your body's mechanisms with exogeneous hormones, new and often unforeseen issues can arise. While gender affirmation via hormones is generally considered safe, and while the benefits for most transgender individuals far outweigh the risks, this process should always be undertaken under a doctor's supervision.

Unfortunately, this isn't always what happens. While the medical environment is becoming friendlier to transgender persons, many who don't have the support of family or community still attempt to transition on their own, using hormone "kits" available on the internet. These medications may be altered or diluted by unscrupulous sellers or may simply not be the right brand, dose, or combination for specific individuals and their unique health concerns. I understand that, for those without adequate social support, insurance, funds, or other resources, transitioning without medical supervision often feels like the only way; for many, the reality of depression, self-harm, or even suicidal thoughts is too much to bear, despite the dangers of self-directed transition. However, as a doctor, I feel compelled to reiterate that the risk of unforeseen complications throughout the process of gender reassignment is already great in a multitude of areas, and it increases exponentially when steps are undertaken without medical supervision.

This isn't meant to instill any fear around gender transition or to discourage people from affirming their gender; in fact, quite the opposite. It's simply important to be aware of and vigilantly monitor the effects and changes that exogenous hormones precipitate. Also, because we have so little information about what happens when someone uses gender-altering hormones long-term, it's important if you're in transition (or if someone you love is in that process) to work closely with providers you trust on a long-term basis to make sure you identify and minimize any issues as soon as they arise.

It's also important to note that transgender people are far more likely than any other population group to be subject to implicit bias, so whether you're considering gender reassignment, currently in transition, or fully transitioned, it's vitally important to find doctors' offices, hospitals, and care facilities at which you feel comfortable, respected, and secure. As you've learned throughout this book, physicians need the right information in order to provide the right care; it's therefore often necessary to share details like birth sex, gender identity, current hormone prescriptions and doses, and which organs are still present (if you've undergone sex reassignment surgery) with one or more providers in the course of both routine and emergency care. For example, if you are a transgender male but still have your uterus and ovaries, you're still at risk for things like ovarian cysts and uterine fibroids. If you need to go to the hospital for abdominal pain, it's important for your providers to know this so they can more accurately diagnose your condition. It may also be necessary in certain situations for you to be seen unclothed. Therefore, it's essential to identify in advance where you want to receive care, and from whom, and to work to build a relationship of trust with your providers. If you don't feel that you are being treated equally with other patients for *any* reason, find another doctor or facility. Period.

Of note for transgender patients is the LGBT Foundation's Pride in Practice programme. This initiative aims to strengthen and develop Primary Care Services' relationships with their lesbian, gay, bisexual and transgender patients in the Greater Manchester area through quality assurance and reporting.

Taking It Home

The female body is highly complex, and adding exogenous hormones to the mix can both relieve common symptoms and create additional complications and side effects ranging from minor to dangerous.

If you are taking any type of exogenous hormones—whether for birth control, menopausal symptoms, support for other medications, or gender affirmation—it's important to communicate with your providers on an ongoing basis to monitor potential side effects and make sure that you're using the lowest appropriate dose. If you are experiencing unwanted side effects, another brand of hormones or a different dose or combination may be better for you. Also, if you add or remove other prescriptions, you may also need to adjust the dose of hormones you're taking.

It's also important to weigh the risks of using exogenous hormones against the benefits. For example, if you are taking HRT for bone-loss prevention but are more than ten years past menopause, the risk of heart disease, dementia, and breast cancer may be higher for you and may outweigh the benefits. If you're on oral birth control but also smoke, are obese, have a preexisting clotting condition, or routinely take long flights, it may be helpful to discuss other pregnancy-prevention options with your doctor.

Also, if your current hormone prescription is producing side effects for you, don't assume that you need to live with them! There may be a better approach; whether it's a shift in dosing, a new generic, or a different combination of prescriptions, your provider may be able to find a better solution for you. Sometimes just opening a discussion can lead to a solution you couldn't foresee previously.

What Matters—Your Key Takeaways

- Women take exogenous hormones for many reasons every day, including for birth control, hormone replacement, and gender affirmation. These hormones are also found in non-oral birth control such as IUDs, implantable devices, and transdermal patches.

- If you are a cisgender or trans woman, taking exogenous hormones for birth control, HRT, or other purposes can increase your risk of DVT, pulmonary embolism, clotting disorders, and stroke. This risk is increased if you smoke, are obese, or have preexisting pulmonary or circulatory conditions.

- While hormone replacement therapies have come a long way and can be effective in many areas, risk factors are still present. Women need to understand these risks so they can make appropriate decisions and be aware of potential complications.

- Transgender individuals often take exogenous hormones for gender affirmation. Hormones that affirm a person's gender may also put trans people at risk for certain conditions associated with that biological sex, particularly with regard to circulatory and cardiac conditions, and may also cause changes in brain patterns and mood.

- Regardless of how or why you are taking exogenous hormones, it's vital to have an open dialogue with your trusted providers to ensure that side effects and risks are minimized and that hormone dosages are adapted to meet your changing needs.

- If you are having a reaction to a specific drug or are experiencing side effects from your exogenous hormones, don't assume that you need to live with this! Ask for a different formulation, a different class of drug, or a new generic. Chances are, there is a better solution for you.

chapter eight

A NEW PERCEPTION: GENDER, CULTURE, AND IDENTITY MEDICINE

We witnessed a sad and traumatic scene recently in my ED.

A family was involved in an awful car crash while driving in their minivan. Three young children were injured, one adult needed an emergency operation to repair internal bleeding, and the grand-mother, who was in the passenger's seat, was fatally injured.

During trauma situations, when standard CPR isn't possible because of injuries to the ribs or lungs, excessive bleeding, or punc-ture wounds, we will sometimes perform what's called a resuscita-tive thoracotomy, where we cut open a person's chest cavity, spread the ribs, and physically massage the heart to keep it beating while we look for internal bleeding and attempt other lifesaving repairs.

Thoracotomies are extreme and are only done as a last resort, and only when the patient has no other chance of survival. They only work in about 1 percent of blunt trauma cases, but I've seen a few patients almost miraculously restored to life when nothing else could have saved them.

Unfortunately, this grandmother was not one of those miracle cases and eventually succumbed to her injuries. It was heartbreaking for all of us—especially the resident on duty, who hadn't encountered a multiple-trauma situation like this outside the classroom.

As the family gathered, the resident encountered something else he hadn't experienced firsthand: cultural beliefs about death that differed from his own. The resident had been raised Catholic, and the family was Muslim; in some conservative Muslim families, men and women are separated in their roles after a death.

When someone dies in the ED, we clean the body as best we can and bring it to a designated room where family and friends can gather and say good-bye. When the resident began to enter that room to offer his condolences to the grandmother's family, he was kindly but firmly asked to leave, as the family's faith practice allowed only women near the grandmother's body now that she had passed on.

As with Jewish custom, an important part of Muslim practice around death is that the body be interred as soon as possible. The body is traditionally buried without a casket so that it may return to the earth as part of a holistic cycle.[1] In this situation, this meant that the medical examiner needed to be called in the middle of the night to perform the standard postmortem examination rather than waiting until morning. And since the family preferred that only women touch the grandmother's body, they requested that the medical examiner be a woman. (Luckily, the examiner on call was female.)

In an emergency setting, some family or religious traditions can be unfamiliar to attending staff and, as such, can seem at odds with "standard" protocol. When medical staff are unprepared for or under-educated about them, this can create friction and misunderstandings.

The resident who'd been on the scene discussed this afterward with me.

"I'm glad we were able to accommodate the family," he said. "I was surprised when they asked me to leave—but I get it now. I just wish I'd known beforehand how to navigate the situation. I mean, what would have happened if the medical examiner on call was male, or if we hadn't had a female doctor on this shift?"

"Those are great questions," I replied. "And we can't always expect to have all the answers. Honestly, the best we can do is be conscious of what we don't know."

As in most cases where there is no existing "rule book," it's our job as providers to take all the information into account and come up with the best possible solution in the moment. In situations like the one I just described, many different social, cultural, and personal preferences and feelings are at play. I feel like it's my job to reinforce to the residents I teach that it's more important to see and hear our patients and their families than it is to have all the answers all the time.

However, such situations are also places where the inherent biases of our medical system are revealed. Our postmortem practices are designed to dovetail with a modern Christian model, wherein the body is refrigerated, embalmed, and eventually buried in a casket or cremated. Our examination practices are designed with the protocols and modesty standards of white, Western people in mind. And, as you've learned thus far in this book, our entire medical system is designed to cater to male bodies and male disease patterns—specifically, white male bodies and white male diseases. This is a recipe for inequality.

A medical model and system that has, historically, used white male bodies almost exclusively as the baseline for all its research, protocol design, and education is going to be biased. There's no way around it. Perpetuating this is the fact that, even today, the majority of doctors and researchers are white—about 72 percent of direct patient/primary care physicians, according to a recent study, with only slightly more diversity across the specialties.[2]

And while everyone who works in medicine—from doctors and nurses to technicians and administrative staff—brings his or her own set of cultural, racial, and religious experiences and ideas, the bigger issue, in my mind, is the medical industry itself. It's a labyrinth of systems and information, but it's like a tower leaning to one side, because all its foundational protocols are based on a male-centric model. We've unintentionally codified sex, gender, and racial inequities in everything from research to staffing to patient care processes, because diversity wasn't taken into account when these things were being developed decades ago. When it comes to some core practices—like what happens after someone dies in the hospital—we're still operating on the same model we were following in the 1980s.

And while, in my experience, most people who work in the medical field are genuinely concerned with the well-being of their patients regardless of race or culture, our system does, unfortunately, provide a platform to amplify the unconscious biases of individuals, simply because it's so heavily skewed toward white, male norms.

My resident's questions really drove home for me our lack of protocol regarding culture, race, and gender differences. Until we start teaching sensitive and unbiased ways of practicing, unintentional conflicts and misunderstandings will continue to arise.

We have hundreds of internal checkpoints and systems in place in the ED to ensure that everything is attended to and no balls are dropped, especially in high-stress situations. When religion and culture clash with these protocols, it's up to the providers on the scene to work with patients and families. Most will, and gladly—but I know that over the years there have been similar situations in hospitals around the country where individual providers have handled things with less than full consideration. Unfortunately, they have been supported by our system in doing so because, on paper, they were "just following the rules."

Medicine in Color

It's impossible to talk about sex and gender in medicine without touching on race, ethnicity, and cultural identity. However, it's vital to understand that, while sex and genetics are biological factors, race—much like gender—is a social construct.[3] This means that perceptions of gender roles and racial "differences" are the product of social and behavioral conditioning, rather than of anything we can measure using scientific methods, and that as a result they vary from culture to culture.

As we've been learning throughout this book, women are understudied, undertreated, and underdiagnosed in medicine as a whole. But within the female population, other groups are even less studied and are repeatedly shown to have even poorer outcomes in multiple key areas.

For example, black, Latina, Muslim, and indigenous American women all experience statistically staggering differences in morbidity, mortality, and treatment outcomes when compared to white women. In fact, the Robert Wood Johnson Foundation estimated that Latino people experienced 30 to 40 percent poorer health outcomes than whites.[4] Black women are three to four times more likely to die in childbirth,[5] 50 percent more likely to die of breast cancer, 50 percent less likely to be treated when they arrive at a hospital with symptoms of heart attack or coronary disease,[6] and 30 percent more likely to die of heart disease than white women—and these are just the tip of the iceberg when it comes to statistics. On the whole, women of color are consistently less likely than white women to receive appropriate treatment in all medical settings, especially when it comes to pain and nonspecific symptoms—like those that, as we've learned, frequently precede female heart attack and stroke or accompany autoimmune and pain disorders.

This is due in part to the unconscious and often generational biases that providers carry with regard to who women of color are, how they behave, and how they communicate. For example, there are pervasive myths that black people have "thicker skin" and therefore feel less pain; this fallacy, along with other cultural myths about race, is apparently believed and acted upon by up to 40 percent of first-year medical students, according to a recent study.[7] (Thankfully, that number is cut by half or more by the time those students get to residency, but the numbers certainly don't zero out.) Cambodian women are considered unusually stoic; the collective belief is that if these women come to the hospital seeking treatment, there must be something *really* wrong, so we should pull out all the stops. On the other hand, women from Central and South America are considered more prone to drama and exaggeration. (Remember my story about "status Hispanicus" from Chapter 6?)

Now, I want to be clear: I study race, culture, and identity issues where they intersect with sex and gender in medical settings, but I'm not a specialist in racial matters in medicine. My focus is on biology and on the social determinants of health directly related to biological sex. Therefore, I can't speak with authority to the root causes and cultural origins of gender- and race-related problems, the specific ways in which they play out on a person-to-person basis across the medical world, or how factors like socioeconomics and location feed into quality of care. I *can* say, however, both clinically and anecdotally, that regardless of where the stereotypes come from and how individual medical personnel embrace or deny them, our male-centric system serves women of color more poorly than it does any other group of people (except, perhaps, the trans-community, but no study has been carried out on that yet).

There are many reasons for this, a great number of which have to do with access to quality care. As one article published by Brookings observed, "African Americans are disproportionately treated at health care facilities with the fewest technological resources, the most poorly trained professionals, and [the] least experienced clinicians." In general, Latina and black women are less likely to receive the regular care and screenings that help identify diseases like cancer early on, in part because many communities lack access to adequate facilities.

However, even the glaring issues in access don't account for the disparities in outcomes for women of color.

As I shared in Chapter 3, many key studies in clinical research and pharmaceutical development include only a small number of women in general, let alone women of color. This leaves us with very little information on which to base our clinical decisions; we simply don't understand what role racial genetics play in key processes like pharmacokinetics and disease development. We need more information in order to understand why some of our most common medical treatments work less well for women of color—and we need that information to go over and above the information we already need to gather about women in general.

Another factor that I believe plays an important role in how women of color receive care is communication. Even barring an actual language barrier, women of color often don't feel heard or understood by their providers. This can happen whether or not the provider carries his or her own implicit bias—but when bias is present, it obviously amplifies the problem.

As we learned in Chapter 6, the "amplification effect" comes into play in many situations between women and their providers, particularly when it comes to pain. This factor is even more of an issue for women of color when racial bias is at play.

When women feel that their providers are ambivalent (or even antagonistic) toward them based on ingrained judgments and prejudices, they are less likely to communicate, which further impedes and obstructs their care. Studies show that black and Latina women are less likely to seek care for fear that they won't be believed or that they'll be endangered by biased or uncaring medical staff. There are plenty of awful stories circulating in the media that underscore this legitimate fear.

There's also research evidence to suggest that the communication issue may be compounded by something called "stereotype threat."[8] This is a disruptive psychological state experienced when people feel like they are the receiving end of a negative stereotype about their cultural identity and are concerned that their behavior might reinforce that image. Basically, it feels like the person is "walking on eggshells," trying to preempt judgment or confirmation of biases—and as a result, their cognitive performance and communication skills are negatively impacted. This phenomenon has been found to contribute to the score gap between white children and minorities in our educational system and also plays out between patients and providers. Women of color should know that it's not their fault if they feel challenged about communicating their symptoms while simultaneously attempting to police their behavior in order to avoid judgment from providers; this is stereotype threat in action.

Diversity Is the Answer

I hear frequently from my black, Latina, and Asian colleagues, friends, and patients that it often feels like the bias in our medical system is insurmountable. However, new research on diversity and inclusivity in medicine is providing some hope that many of these problems can be alleviated, even within our current male-centric system.[9]

The first thing we all need to do, of course, is to police our own assumptions. Providers may be making decisions about how they treat women of color based in unconscious biases or even faulty information. Such judgments precede every interaction; unless and until we are aware of them, individually and collectively, they will continue to negatively affect the level of care women receive in all medical settings.

I've been asking the residents and attending physicians with whom I work questions like, "Where do you see bias playing out against women in general or women of color in particular?" One of my colleagues shared with me a simple story that provided a clinical example of unconscious bias.

When I asked her, "Where do you see bias at play in the ED?" she immediately answered, "The first thing that comes to mind is chronic abdominal pain."

Women are more likely to have unexplained chronic abdominal pain, so when a female patient comes in with this kind of complaint, providers are less likely to order heavy-duty tests. "I have a lower suspicion that I'll get a positive diagnosis," my colleague said.

As fate would have it, a patient came into the ED later that night with chronic abdominal pain. When my colleague finished the exam, she sought me out. "I've been thinking about what you asked me all day. This patient has a history of kidney stones, so I ordered an ultrasound. But I just realized that, if she'd been a man, I would have ordered a CT scan."

"Why do you say that?" I asked.

She shook her head. "I can't believe I'm admitting bias to you! But honestly, I had to catch myself. I was assuming that it was going to turn out to be nothing, so I ordered the least invasive test possible and figured we'd go from there."

There is clinical reasoning at play here, of course. CT scans deliver a substantial dose of radiation and should be utilized judiciously. Kidney stones often show up on an ultrasound, so the primary concern for the patient was in fact being addressed. But the fact remains that if the patient had been male, a different diagnostic pathway might have been chosen.

If we are to stay true to the Hippocratic oath many of us swore when we graduated from medical school, we need to be aware of where individual and collective biases may be rearing their heads in our day-to-day work. As one translation of the oath reads, "I will remember that I remain a member of society, with special obligations to all my fellow human beings, those sound of mind and body as well as the infirm."[10]

The second thing we can do to increase equality of care is to create a path into medical fields that is open to all. As I shared earlier, the majority of doctors in America are still white and male.[11] (In the United Kingdom and Europe, the percentage of female doctors is higher, but physicians are still overwhelmingly white.)[12] And while women are now overtaking men in certain specialties (such as reproductive health), and while people of color represent a growing segment of medical school graduates, the diversity of the medical field does not remotely correlate to the diversity of our country's population.

It's been observed that patient care improves with gender and racial congruence. A study conducted in Oakland, California, recently demonstrated this in action.[13] Researchers enrolled more than 1,300 black men from barbershops across the city (the idea being that since everyone gets haircuts, they could select a wide range of ages, health statuses, and income levels for the study population). They then created a clinic staffed by six black and eight nonblack doctors to serve participants. Patients were then given surveys and offered incentives to show up for preventive care services. The results were telling: while initially patients selected the same number of preventive care services regardless of the race of their provider, over time, only the men seeing black doctors utilized more preventive services than initially agreed. These effects were most pronounced for men who initially stated a mistrust of the medical system.

These findings make clear that when people trust and can comfortably communicate with their providers, they are more likely to engage in the kind of preventative care that reduces disease and creates more positive long-term outcomes.

However, despite the evidence that racial congruence improves outcomes, this is *not* an argument for striating patients according of the race of the provider or even for simply bringing more doctors of color to underserved or primarily minority communities. Instead, it's a case for greater diversity in *all* facilities to invite a factor I call "collective intelligence."

Studies show that when physicians operate in a space where their colleagues are of diverse sex, race, and ethnic backgrounds, the quality of care for *all* patients—including people of color and women—improves.[14] For example, a large-scale, long-term study conducted in Florida found that female heart attack patients had measurably worse outcomes when they were treated by male physicians versus female physicians—but that their outcomes improved markedly when (1) the male physicians had extensive experience treating female patients and (2) the male physicians had many female colleagues.[15] Basically, male doctors who work closely with women do a better job treating their female patients.

Other studies have demonstrated this effect across the spectrum of race. A combination of a diverse workplace, cultural competence among physicians, and elevated interpersonal communication skills (which themselves are enhanced by a diverse work environment) consistently results in better quality of care, particularly for black patients.[16] Trust and consistency was another key factor in leveling the field; this was demonstrated in a 2008 report by researchers at George Washington University titled *Racial and Ethnic Disparities in U.S. Health Care: A Chartbook*.[17] The authors noted that when people of color have a "medical home"—meaning providers in a single location whom they can see and communicate with regularly and grow to trust—"the percentage of patients who receive needed medical care increases across all groups and racial and ethnic disparities are virtually eliminated."

Steps are being taken within medical institutions to close the gap and address the issues of implicit and explicit bias. My colleague Sheryl L. Heron, MD, MPH, FACEP, coauthored a medical textbook dedicated to the ideas of cultural competency and diversity, titled *Diversity and Inclusion in Quality Patient Care*.[18] Hospitals and medical centers, particularly teaching hospitals, are including such training for staff at all levels. But the best solution, in my mind, is still to create a medical environment where the doctors, nurses, and staff are as diverse as their patients—an environment where everyone is seen, heard, and represented.

As my colleague Esther K. Choo, MD, succinctly noted in a recent presentation, "It's reasonable to say that a heterogeneous physician population is a better fit for our heterogeneous patient population."

Taking It Home

If you are a woman of color or have experienced implicit or explicit bias with regard to your religious or cultural beliefs, you don't have to stay silent or avoid medical treatment while those of us within the system work to create change. There are choices you can make right now to improve your quality of care, be seen and heard, and become part of the push for equality within the medical system.

The most powerful thing you can do is to choose providers whom you trust and by whom you feel heard. Research doctors and facilities in your area. Don't be afraid to interview potential providers! Most primary care physicians will schedule a "meet and greet" appointment where you can essentially interview them about their practice. If you don't like what you're hearing or seeing, find someone else.

If you have a choice of hospitals in your area, look for those that provide cultural competence and/or diversity and inclusion training to their staff, have a diverse staff of doctors and nurses, and have a good social track record for working with diverse populations. While you may not always be able to choose your individual provider in an emergency situation, you are likely to receive better care when collective intelligence is at play.[19]

If you are in an end-of-life situation and would like to make sure your family's spiritual practices are understood and accommodated, involve a spiritual care provider from your hospital. You may have been asked upon arrival about your faith and how you would like certain situations addressed; a spiritual care provider can act as an advocate for you with hospital staff.[20]

And finally, if you're dealing with a specific condition or set of healthcare challenges, it may be helpful to join a solutions-focused support group. You can also investigate how to add your voice to the conversation by participating in local studies, surveys, and other research projects.

Most of all, remember that you're not imagining things; there really does exist both explicit and implicit bias in medicine. However, most individual providers really do want to do their best for their patients. As a woman of color, you can still get great care no matter what the race or gender of your physician, but you will absolutely want to have an open and honest conversation about your experiences within the medical system, your concerns about bias, and your unique healthcare needs. As studies have shown and as I've shared in this chapter, trust and communication are the biggest factors in making sure that women of all ethnicities and backgrounds get the best possible care.

In the end, it's not the job of women of color to educate their providers on implicit bias or racial disparities. It's on us in the medical world to educate ourselves, call out bias where we see it (even in ourselves), and do better for our diverse patient population. But as we work toward that goal, individually and institutionally, maintaining open lines of communication is key.

Your voice matters. The medical world needs to hear it.

What Matters—Your Key Takeaways

- Racial bias in medicine happens both at the level of individual providers and systemically. This is in part because of existing bias on an individual level and in part because our entire medical system was designed around a white, male model.

- The systems at play in medical settings are often at odds with cultural traditions and mandates. Communication is key to making sure your beliefs are honored.

- Patients statistically receive better care when there is gender and/or racial congruence between patient and provider and also at facilities where there is a diverse mix of doctors and staff.

- Many hospitals are now mandating diversity and inclusion training, as well as cultural competence certifications, for doctors, nurses, and other staff. If you have a choice of hospitals, ask whether staff are being educated as to how to better serve you.

WHERE WE'RE HEADED—AND WHAT YOU CAN DO

chapter nine

A CHANGING CONVERSATION: THE FUTURE OF SEX AND GENDER RESEARCH IN MEDICINE

In 2012, my colleague Esther K. Choo, MD, and I were approached by Basmah Safdar, MD, director of the Yale New Haven Hospital Chest Pain Center, and Marna Greenberg, DO, director of emergency medicine research at Lehigh Valley Hospital, about a collaboration.

"Let's put together something to present on sex and gender medicine at the SAEM Consensus Conference," they said. Of course, Dr. Choo and I were honored to be invited to collaborate.

We spent nearly a year creating a hefty proposal and presentation plan for this highly competitive conference and, several months later, found out that we'd been accepted.

In 2014, over one hundred top emergency medicine researchers showed up for our daylong symposium. We looked at cardio- and cerebrovascular issues, pain, trauma and injury, diagnostic imaging, mental health, and substance abuse through the lens of sex and gender. We also touched on social perceptions and how they influence our in-the-moment choices in the emergency department.

That day, we created one hundred new experts in sex and gender medicine. Since then, that number has grown exponentially—and Drs. Choo, Safdar, and Greenberg have become long-term friends and collaborators.

In 2015, I helped to design and facilitate an event titled "Sex and Gender Medicine Education Summit: A Roadmap for Curricular Innovation." This collective initiative of the American Medical Women's Association, the Laura Bush Institute for Women's Health, the Mayo Clinic, and the Society for Women's Health Research was held on the campus of the Mayo Clinic. Our more than 170 in-person and virtual attendees represented faculty and deans from ninety-nine U.S. medical schools, as well as federal agencies and research organizations. Over the course of the two-day symposium, we provided information and tools to begin to integrate sex-differences research into medical school curricula and ongoing education programs for providers.

Then, in April 2018, we expanded our platform via the Sex and Gender Health Education Summit in Salt Lake City, Utah. This opened the doors for educators in all health professions—including dentistry, nursing, pharmacy, and "allied health" professions like physical therapy and occupational therapy—to learn how to integrate sex-differences research into their educational curricula and create a step-by-step plan for sex and gender integration. A similar event was co-hosted by the BMA and Medical Women's Federation in London in November 2019.

Every time we bring a group of professionals together in a setting like these, it facilitates a wave of change. It's my mission to keep those waves coming—to create a tide of change and eventually a tsunami. Ultimately, I know, we will reach a tipping point where what was once unusual and specialized will become common knowledge and practice.

Change at the Educational and Administrative Levels

In Chapter 2, I shared that, when I put together my first talk on sex and gender in emergency medicine for the SAEM conference, no one showed up. That empty room was definitely discouraging—but it also strengthened my resolve to get the message out there.

After that day, I decided to reach out to other women in the medical field who were having similar conversations. I ended up going to the American Medical Women's Association, where I connected with Janice Werbinski, MD, FACOG, NCMP, who is an associate clinical professor emerita in obstetrics and gynecology (OB/GYN) at the Western Michigan University Homer R. Stryker M.D. School of Medicine. We started talking about how we could create an interdisciplinary "think tank"—a forum to discuss and disseminate ideas about sex and gender issues in medicine, then take those ideas back to our individual specialties.

Those initial conversations were the foundation of what would become the Sex and Gender Women's Health Collaborative (SGWHC). Dr. Werbinski has tirelessly led this organization and remains its executive director. At first, we were simply holding monthly conference calls with a core group of six to eight women—but soon, it began to grow and eventually became the organization and resource it is today.

It was on one of those initial calls that I connected with Marjorie R. Jenkins, MD, FACP, a tenured professor of medicine at Texas Tech University Health Sciences Center. She was one of the first women to really make "women's health" about sex and gender rather than merely reproduction, and I'd looked up to her for a long time. She is such a presence; when she speaks, people really listen. On one phone call, M.J. (as I call her) shared that two of the posters we'd created through the SGWHC had been accepted for display at the annual Organization for the Study of Sex Differences conference. Someone would need to stand under the posters during the event and speak to attendees about the work we were doing.

"I can't stand in two places at once," M.J. said. "So who's coming with me?"

I was only a junior physician at the time, but I immediately volunteered. I would have to fly in that morning and fly home the same night in order to be there for my shift at the hospital the next morning, but I didn't care. I wanted to show this amazing woman that I was a doer and that I was serious.

Turns out, the posters were displayed next to one another at the event, so for the two-hour session, M.J. and I stood together and spoke to other medical professionals about the importance of sex and gender differences across all specialties. Between conversations, she and I spoke about what we believed needed to happen in medicine and science to bring women's outcomes up to par. From then on, we've been friends and collaborators. Even now, when we get together, we can't stop talking about sex and gender issues. It's nice to have someone who not only shares my passion for creating change but is leading the charge in her own field.

Today, Dr. Jenkins serves as the founding director and chief scientific officer of the Laura Bush Institute for Women's Health, where she has significantly advanced sex- and gender-specific education within the medical field. The institute has developed a curriculum for practitioners—including modules to help educate future educators, to which I've been honored to contribute. It also has a library of resources for laypeople that is free and accessible to everyone.

Many more wonderful organizations are on the cutting edge of change in medical education and research. I can't name them all here, but I do want to call attention to several around the world whose work continues to create a dramatic positive impact on medical education as a whole.

One fantastic initiative is actually taking place at the time of this writing within the National Institutes of Health (NIH). Led by Janine Clayton, MD, the Office for Research on Women's Health (ORWH)—one of twenty-seven individual institutes and centers (ICs) within the organization—has created an initiative called the Trans-NIH Strategic Plan for Women's Health Research to advance research relevant to the health of women and enhance implementation of data and evidence to improve women's health. Rather than try to do it all with its limited office budget, the ORWH created an NIH-wide initiative to include sex and gender research in the studies and funding of *all* the organization's ICs. This not only increases the ORWH's reach but also means that nearly all the research funded by the NIH is now encouraged or even required to include metrics for sex differences. This is a huge step forward in multiple areas and will certainly provide us with a vast body of new information that we can use to improve women's outcomes in all areas of medicine. I'm honored to have been asked to serve on the advisory board of the ORWH in 2019.

The Food and Drug Administration (FDA) also has an Office of Women's Health, which is working to increase sex and gender equality and increase awareness and advocacy. This office was the force behind the FDA's Drug Trials Snapshots resource I shared in Chapter 4. Unfortunately, this office lacks the power to mandate—so it can't, for example, force pharmaceutical companies to include sex-specific metrics in drug trials—but it is creating helpful resources, encouraging transparency, and starting necessary conversations.

At Stanford University, the Gendered Innovations program, led by Londa Schiebinger, PhD, focuses on sex-specific analysis in the fields of science, health, engineering, and environment. It is working with things like gendered crash-test dummies and female artificial intelligence programs and introducing the use of gendered cells in scientific and medical research. As the program's website says, "Doing research right can save lives and money."

And the Barbra Streisand Women's Heart Center at Cedars-Sinai, where my colleague C. Noel Bairey Merz, MD, is the director, is pioneering research into sex-specific diagnoses and treatment of female-pattern heart disease, including Takotsubo's and small vessel disease.

Internationally, big things are happening in sex and gender research as well. The Canadian Institutes of Health Research includes the Institute of Gender and Health. That office's scientific director, Cara Tannenbaum, MD, MSc, is working not only to bring sex differences into research across Canada but also to study gender differences in both medical settings and society at large. Her office has online training modules for physicians and providers about how to incorporate sex and gender into both research and clinical practice. It's very well done and highly inclusive.

The Charité Hospital at the Universitätsmedizin Berlin is also on the leading edge of sex and gender protocols. They've successfully implemented e-training modules and a vast literature database featuring the research into the field of gender in medicine, which studies mainly biological sex differences including cellular and molecular mechanisms.

In Sweden, the Karolinska Institute has developed an interdisciplinary teaching resource and research platform to promote sex and gender awareness. Its "Four I's" represent the four pillars of its approach: infrastructure, integration, innovation, and impact. The institute collaborates with renowned organizations worldwide, including the Mayo Clinic in the United States, the Gendered Innovations program at Stanford University referenced earlier, and EUGenMed (European Gender Medicine, a group overseen by Charité and the European Institute of Women's Health).

Saving Lives Through Simple Tools

While changing the medical curriculum and worldwide research protocol is vital to educating the next generation of doctors and providers, it's a long-term plan. We also need boots-on-the-ground tools to help women get the health care they need today.

In my own emergency department at Rhode Island Hospital, as well as in the national and international conversation currently taking place about sex and gender in medicine, there's a constant thought process happening around simple but effective ways to create impactful results with regard to women's health and sex differences.

In my own ED, we employ strategies like "We Know the Difference" posters and patient information pamphlets, as well as complex and multilayered in-person and video training for interns, residents, fellows, nurses, and faculty. Similar trainings, many of which I've helped to develop, are taking place across the country, so that providers can become aware of and adapt to the flood of new information available about how women's bodies operate and what we can do to provide better outcomes across the full spectrum of women's health.

But perhaps the most powerful innovations we as a medical community have engineered over the last several years are changes to common treatment protocols.

It's been recognized for a long time that decision support tools—basically, checklists of procedures and protocols—in operating rooms save lives and decrease complications. There are checklists for everything from making sure you have the right patient and are doing surgery on the correct side of the body to counting instruments and surgical sponges to make sure nothing was left inside the patient. But recently, some researchers have been creating decision support tools with the intention of equalizing outcomes between men and women.

For example, as I noted earlier in this book, it's known that women, especially women who use birth control, are at higher risk of blood clots than men of similar ages. However, it's also true that women are less likely to receive prophylaxis (aka, preventive treatment) for numerous considerations, including blood clots, after a trauma surgery. Such preventive measures might include injections to prevent clotting or the use of special stockings to prevent deep vein thrombosis in the limbs. (Thrombosis is correlated with immobility and, in particular, with hospital stays. On average, nearly 30,000 hospitalized adults die each year from complications due to venous thromboembolism [VTE].)

So why, when all this is known, are women statistically less likely to receive prophylaxis for clotting? Doctors at Johns Hopkins University asked the same question. As an experiment, they created a decision support tool for people coming out of surgery who were at risk of clotting complications.[1] When this protocol was followed, researchers found that "risk-appropriate VTE prophylaxis increased from 26% to 80% for surgical patients and from 25% to 92% for medical patients." Making a simple decision support tool a mandatory part of daily hospital protocol saved literally hundreds of lives.

The Cleveland Clinic conducted a similar experiment with regard to ST-elevation myocardial infarction (the "widow maker" condition that my patient Julie from Chapter 1 experienced). They found that when a standard four-step protocol was followed, women's thirty-day risk of mortality was reduced by half—from 6 to 3 percent. More important, this reduction put their risk on par with that of men. And the only thing that had changed was the delivery of care.

This shows us that implicit bias can be alleviated, and deadly complications avoided, when we implement comprehensive systems based on the latest research and data. These systems are sometimes complex to design, but when well organized and put into regular use, they can streamline the daily workflow of doctors, nurses, and technicians, as well as improve the outcomes of patients.

My Vision for the Future of Medicine

When we mapped the human genome, the medical community at large was sure that personalized medicine would be the next big breakthrough. Everything from cancer treatments to heart disease prevention, it was dreamed, would be based on individual genetic criteria and information. Soon there would be a pill for every person, and we would finally conquer what is killing us.

Unfortunately, the reality turned out to be far more complex than we could have imagined. Genes alone aren't what determines disease. And even when they are, we aren't even close to understanding the multifaceted processes by which genes are turned on or off. We thought we had conquered a pond; instead, we have plunged into an ocean.

I'm a huge proponent of research into personalized medicine, but I also recognize that we are a long way away from the vision that researchers originally conceived. And, quite honestly, we can't get there from here. How can we develop and implement truly personalized medicine until we acknowledge the difference between male and female biology, bring that knowledge into every research model and clinical protocol, and use what we learn as first-phase building blocks for personalizing treatment? In some respects, we're trying to go from the basement to the penthouse without stopping to do the work on the floors between.

I envision a future in which medical treatment is highly personalized according to biological sex *and* preferred gender, as well as genetic ethnicity and ancestry. But in order to get there, we need to start with the basics. We need to redesign our male-centric system so that women are treated according to their own separate and distinct biology. We need to study the genetic structures within both male and female ethnic and ancestral groups, as well as the social constructs of race and gender, so that we can provide equal and effective care to women from all walks of life.

I imagine a system where pharmaceuticals and treatments are sex-specific, where we have separate dosing strategies for men and women for all drugs available. I imagine detailed dosing guidelines for women at various points in their menstrual cycles, for women in the peri- and postmenopausal phases of life, for women on certain types of birth control, and for women who are pregnant. I imagine unique decision support tools for male and female patients and laboratory values consistent with what's normal for female bodies, not just male ones.

I imagine mandatory trainings for all medical professionals in the areas of gender relationships, inclusion, cultural competence, and diversity. I imagine the implementation of system-wide protocols to minimize the ways in which bias can play out in patient-provider interactions. I imagine outcomes for women of color, transgender persons, and women of diverse religions becoming equal to those of white men.

Most of all, I imagine better care across the board for *all* women, in all settings, and across all stages of life.

These are the things that will transform medicine. And the best way to make them a reality is to start with the broad reality of sex differences and work our way in.

What Matters—Your Key Takeaways

- Sex and gender differences are a hot topic in medicine today. Many important institutions and organizations, including at the federal level, are working to change research and clinical practice standards to reflect our new knowledge of female biology.
- The most important places to facilitate changes are in educational curricula, research, and clinical practice guidelines. Of those, clinical practice guidelines can be implemented most quickly.
- The future of personalized medicine begins with sex-differences research. What we learn there will pave the way to greater understanding of the way individual bodies work.

chapter ten

YOUR VOICE, YOUR MEDICINE: HOW TO HAVE HELPFUL CONVERSATIONS WITH YOUR PROVIDERS

THE HARDEST—AND, SIMULTANEOUSLY, the most rewarding—part of my job isn't researching sex and gender differences, or writing articles for peer review, or even educating other providers. It's having productive, outcome-focused conversations with patients and their families.

For example, a woman came into the emergency department recently with a complaint of abdominal pain and blood in her stool. She was very concerned about colon cancer and had made a list of the symptoms she had experienced over the past several days and weeks. She was up front about her history of irritable bowel disease, constipation, and other gut issues, as well as her frustration that nothing she'd tried in the past seemed to help very much. And, to underscore the conversation, she'd taken a picture of the contents of her toilet to show us.

Unappetizing? A bit. But the fact that she didn't minimize or dance around her symptoms was incredibly helpful. We talked about what she had learned in her Google searches and how long her symptoms had been going on. Her "evidence" showed that the blood was dark, not bright red, so I was able to rule out superficial causes like hemorrhoids or rectal tears and refer her for additional testing. More, I was able to help her feel seen and heard and guide our discussion in a way that let her know that her concerns were being addressed.

Throughout this book, I've made clear the issues in medical practice, research, and education that impact women's health and well-being. I've put forward a call for change and shared some of the research that is driving us toward a new and better understanding of women's unique biology. But, as you've likely surmised, while change *is* happening, it's slow.

The best way for you to shift the conversation around your health and ensure that you receive sex-specific and appropriate care is to have targeted, productive conversations with your providers. In this chapter, I'll give you specific tools and questions to help you do exactly that.

This doesn't mean that the burden of changing the medical system has shifted to you, but it *is* a call for you to become more empowered and vocal around your health and well-being. When you take the reins and use the knowledge you've gained in this book to initiate conversations about your sex and gender in your medical relationships, you will enjoy a feeling of sovereignty over your healthcare choices and pathways.

The New Doctor-Patient Relationship

It's important to remember that, although it often appears otherwise, medicine is in fact a consumer-driven industry. You have choices about what kinds of relationships you want to have with your providers. I think of myself not as an authority figure but rather as a translator of information. My job is to help patients get the help they need in moments of crisis but also to help them make informed decisions that will improve or sustain their health. I know that many, even most, of my colleagues think the same way.

However, like all relationships, the doctor-patient relationship goes both ways. Clear lines of communication are imperative and—whenever possible—need to be established before an emergency situation arises.

That's why I've created the following lists of helpful questions and practices for you to take with you into the most common medical settings and scenarios. Some are basic and apply to everyone, while others are sex and gender specific. As I've mentioned before, knowing how to start and steer the conversation can have powerful and even lifesaving results.

Your Primary Care Provider: The Central Hub of Your Health Care

Your primary care provider (PCP) is more than just the person who does your annual checkup. She or he is like your medical care hub, where all the different pathways of specialists' visits, hospital care, obstetrics and gynecology (OB/GYN), and pharmaceuticals intersect.

Of all the medical providers with whom you interact (or might someday interact), your PCP is by far the most important with whom to develop a trusting, amiable relationship. This is the doctor you will call when something goes wrong but also who will help you heal and maintain your health when things are going well. She or he needs, therefore, to have a clear and accurate picture of your medical history, your current prescriptions, and everything else that's happening with regard to your health.

Your PCP is also the person who will write most of your prescriptions, perform your yearly screenings, and, if necessary, refer you to specialists for testing, surgery, and other procedures.

In other words, you need to trust your PCP's judgment and feel that she or he has your best interests at heart.

If you feel that you are not being seen or heard by your PCP, that you can't be transparent in your discussions, or that you may be on the receiving end of unconscious bias, I encourage you to find a new doctor. It's not that your current PCP isn't great—but in this case, your relationship with your doctor is even more important than that doctor's skill set.

Here are some of the questions you might want to ask your current (or new) PCP on your next visit to ensure that you're getting the best care based on your sex, gender, personal history, and current health situation:

- "What are the latest recommendations for women of my age around…?"
  - Yearly screenings and blood work
  - Breast exams (including mammography)
  - Colonoscopy

- Pap tests
- Other routine testing
- "How often do I need to do the above exams, and why?"
- "Do you perform Pap tests, pelvic exams, and breast exams, or do I need to see my OB/GYN for that?" (Not all PCPs provide these services.)
- "Are you aware of the latest research on sex and gender in your field?"
- "Do you observe that your female patients and patients of color have equal outcomes to your male patients?"

If you live in an area with limited medical facilities, have challenges with transportation, or are underinsured, I encourage you to tap into telemedicine resources like the one developed by my colleague Judd Hollander, MD, at Jefferson University, aptly titled "JeffConnect," which staffs telephones and video call lines with emergency department doctors and specialists.[1] CVS Pharmacy also offers Minute Clinic physician visits through its app. Obviously these resources won't serve you well in a medical emergency, but they are absolutely brilliant for streamlining access to physicians for minor injuries, questions about medications, and preventive care discussions.

Questions for Specialists and Surgeons

Often your PCP will refer to you a specialist for concerns that are beyond her or his purview. Gastroenterologists, endocrinologists, immunologists, and orthopedic surgeons are all examples of specialists.

One thing to remember about specialists: unlike PCPs, they have a narrow and specific focus. And while it's still important to find a specialist you trust and connect with, it's also important to find the best person for the job.

During my residency, I was assigned to a surgical rotation and had the chance to assist several surgeons in multiple disciplines. One surgeon was a particular favorite of patients. He had a great bedside manner, was jovial and positive, and always had time to say hello. He was also the sloppiest surgeon I've ever seen. On the other hand, another surgeon who was incredibly intimidating and impersonal in his patient interactions was absolutely meticulous in the operating room. Sure, I'd rather have a glass of wine with the first guy. But if I was going under the knife, I'd choose doctor number two in a heartbeat.

When meeting a new specialist, a specialist, don't be afraid to ask about outcomes. There's a good chance that those you talk to are involved in some research of their own and will be happy to answer your questions. Here are some to get you started:

- "Have you studied sex differences in your discipline?"
- "Does this test/procedure you're recommending take into account my personal biology?"
- "Have you noticed any disparity in outcomes between your male and female patients?"
- "What are the alternatives if this test doesn't give us the answers we're looking for?"
- "Are there side effects of this test/procedure I should be aware of as a woman?"
- "Will this test/procedure be influenced or impacted by my birth control/pregnancy/breastfeeding/hormone replacement therapy (HRT)?"

Questions About Pharmaceuticals

One of the biggest challenges that I and my colleagues encounter is patients' lack of knowledge about their prescriptions.

In the ED, we don't always have access to patients' full prescription records, especially when patients are getting prescriptions from multiple or out-of-state providers. And when we don't have the whole picture, it's hard to choose the medications that are going to be safest and most effective for that person.

Here are some things you can do to be sure that you can share the whole picture of your prescriptions with any provider who cares for you, both in an emergency setting and elsewhere:

- Compile a complete list of your prescriptions and make sure it's accessible at all times. You don't have to carry a piece of paper in your wallet; our current technology makes this much easier. Just take photos of all of your prescription bottles with your phone's camera and save them to a folder on your phone or in a cloud account where you can easily access them. Make sure the photos are clear enough for someone to read both the prescription name and the dosing information. Update the list once a year or whenever your regimen changes.

- Add your prescriptions and allergy information to your phone's medical ID feature or emergency lock screen. (For instructions about how to do this, visit the website of your phone's maker.) You can also download a free Medical ID app and store all your information there.

- Make sure that at least one of your emergency contacts has access to your up-to-date prescription information. This can be accomplished via a shared cloud drive folder or simply by giving the person a list of your meds once a year when you do your annual update.

- Remember our conversation about medical reconciliation ("Med Rec") in Chapter 4? This is a great time to update your personal medication lists. If you are confused or have questions, especially after a hospital visit (when your prescriptions may have been altered temporarily or permanently), make an appointment with the nurse or physician's assistant in your PCP's office to go over the changes.

Once you have a clear picture of the meds you're taking, you can bring questions like those below to your PCP, as well as any specialist or provider who prescribes you a new medication, adjusts your medication, or oversees your care in a hospital or emergency setting:

- "Are the meds I am taking the right ones for my sex, race/ethnicity, and stage of life?"
- "Am I taking sex-appropriate doses, or do we need to adjust my prescriptions?"
- "Is this medication tested in women? If so, are there different dosing guidelines I should be aware of?"
- "Will this prescription affect my birth control or HRT?"
- "Is this medication a generic, and if so, how might that affect me? Has this generic been studied in women?"
- "Does this medication prolong the QT interval? How might this affect me, given my other medications?"
- "I've observed that I feel different since I started this new generic, and I'm concerned it may not be metabolizing as well as my former medication. Is there another affordable brand I could switch to?"

Hospital and Emergency Visits

Obviously, most people don't plan to visit the ED—and, once there, they don't have much control over who is caring for them. However, there are some simple ways to set the stage for better care and improved outcomes.

The first and most important is to research your local hospitals. Which hospitals in your area have a good reputation? A diverse staff and programs for cultural competence? Which are leading the way in research and education? Don't be afraid to ask questions—or even visit the hospital to talk to the nurses and desk staff! Ask questions about their experience with sex and gender disparities and always "go with your gut."

The second is to be prepared with your information. I love when people come into the ED with detailed descriptions of their symptoms, lists of prescriptions, and a clear grasp of their medical history (even if that means looking at pictures of bowel movements!). Having all the relevant information at hand helps me make the best possible decisions about the patient's care. When people are vague about their medical history (or worse, try to hide parts of it), don't know what prescriptions they're on, or can't describe their symptoms beyond a vague "it hurts here," it is harder for me to help them.

For example, not long ago, an eighty-five-year-old woman named Elise came in on a stretcher. She'd enjoyed a small glass of sangria while at lunch with her girlfriends, but after the check was paid and she went to stand up, she got dizzy and collapsed. When we checked her blood pressure, it was dangerously low.

"Do you know what medications she's on?" I asked the friend who had ridden with her to the ED.

"I don't," she said, shaking her head. "But I can call her daughter."

Thankfully, the daughter had lists of Elise's prescriptions and a clear grasp of her medical history. I discovered that Elise was on several medications for a medical condition that could make alcohol affect her disproportionately. After a brief rest and hydration, Elise was feeling better and ready to go home.

If you are unable to speak when you arrive at the hospital—or even if you're awake but nervous and in pain—having a friend or relative who has access to important information and can communicate it clearly can help us save your life. Here are some things you can do to make sure that, if you do need to be hospitalized, your providers have all the information they need to help you:

- Make sure that at least one friend or family member has access to *all* your medical information, including your prescriptions, recent tests, diagnoses, surgical history, and so forth. List that person as your primary medical contact when you are being registered and be sure that phone number, address, and email information is up to date so we can contact him or her quickly in time-sensitive situations.
- Set up a power of attorney and other legal safeguards to be sure that the person you designate as your advocate can make decisions on your behalf.
- If you are taken to a hospital other than the one you've chosen as your preferred place of care, you can ask to be transferred.
- If you are able, make sure to be transparent about key information on your intake form, such as the following:
  - Allergies—not only what they are but how they manifest, so your doctor can make better decisions around which medications are appropriate. For example, if you have an allergy to an antibiotic, but it's not severe and

only triggers a rash, we might choose to use that medicine anyway in a serious situation. On the other hand, if your reaction is anaphylactic, we need to know that too.

- Family history of disease, including the ages at which your family members were diagnosed. If your mom had a heart attack at eighty-seven, that's a lot less concerning for us than if your mom had a heart attack at forty-seven.
- Any and all hormones that you use, including birth control, HRT, or hormones for gender affirmation.
- Any past or present pregnancy-related complications (such as preeclampsia, gestational diabetes, etc.) that could serve as risk factors for cardiovascular disease.
- Any history of medication reactions.
- Congenital long QT syndrome or other inherited conditions that could impact how medications work in your body.

If You Don't Feel Seen, Heard, or Believed...

Of course, being prepared in advance for a medical situation will help you navigate things with greater confidence and ease. But sometimes, even when you've done everything by the book, you may run into a situation where you feel like gender bias is at play—where you feel like you're not being seen, heard, or believed.

- If you're not in the midst of an emergency, the best thing to do is initiate a conversation and be as specific as possible about what is going on and how you're feeling; however, it's hard to "reset" that crucial patient-provider relationship if it's off-kilter from the start. If you don't feel like you can have a productive conversation with your provider, seek out someone else for a second opinion.

- If you are in a hospital situation, call in an advocate—someone who can give perspective on the situation. For example, an older woman who'd fallen on concrete came in with a subdural hematoma. She insisted she was fine and able to go home—but her sister, whom we'd called when she was brought in, stepped in. "She's such a minimizer. She'd say that even if she could barely walk! Keep her here overnight, please." Since we didn't know this patient, we couldn't have made the correct call without her sister's input.

- Help providers understand that you aren't drug seeking. Unfortunately, opiate addiction is something we deal with on a daily basis in the ED. People come in complaining of subjective conditions like migraine, abdominal pain, or other things we can't observe or measure in order to get OxyContin or Dilaudid. We are actually in the process of creating an integrated prescription monitoring system that tracks opioid prescriptions and administration to prevent abuse of the system. If you are in a lot of pain and feel like you're being treated as a drug seeker, you can ask whether your hospital has a monitoring system and request that your records be referenced to show this isn't the case. (Or if you do have a relationship with opioids via a pain contract with your doctor, you can be transparent about your use and requirements.) You can also state that you aren't seeking any specific drug and are open to nonopioid, nonaddictive pain relief options to address what's happening right now. This isn't meant to put the burden of proof on you or to make it your responsibility to cajole your providers into helping you. But sometimes just knowing you're aware of what they're dealing with can help you shift the conversation with your providers.

- If you feel like the situation can't be improved, ask for a different provider or see if it's possible to be transferred to a different hospital (especially if most of your care has been at that other hospital).

If You Are a Woman of Color...

As we've learned throughout this book, women of color face even more challenges in our medical system than white women. They are less likely to be heard and believed and less likely to receive appropriate treatment than white women.

If you're a woman of color and are concerned about implicit bias or that your religious or ethnic traditions may not be accommodated, you may want to integrate some additional questions into your conversations with your providers. Here are some you might consider:

For individual doctors and specialists:

- "Do you feel that women of color receive the same outcomes as white patients in your practice?"
- "Do you see many women of color in your practice?"
- "Are you willing to hear and discuss my concerns about racial and cultural bias in medical practice?"
- "Are you willing to accommodate [my personal, cultural, or religious concerns] in the course of visits and treatments?"

For hospitals, urgent care centers, and medical groups:

- "Have your doctors and staff received education in cultural competence?"

- "What is your current level of diversity among doctors and staff?"
- "Do you have experience with [your individual cultural/religious practices]? Will you be willing to accommodate my particular requests and concerns?"

The All-Knowing "Doctor Google"

In our current age of information, almost everyone consults "Doctor Google" before making an appointment with a provider.

In many ways, this is a good thing—especially for women. It can help you know what questions to ask and what your symptoms indicate you should be concerned about. You can research your prescriptions, check for drug interactions (especially around your birth control or hormone therapies), and perhaps even discover new information about your prescriptions, your condition, or alternative treatments that even your doctor doesn't know about yet.

I had coffee recently with a med student named Kim who shares a hereditary genetic condition with her twin that results in, among other things, a prolonged QT interval. This condition required both sisters to be on beta blockers starting while they were still in high school. However, after a short time on these drugs, the med student's sister began feeling poorly. Testing revealed that her platelet levels were falling rapidly.

"I did some research on my own," Kim shared, "and found out that the beta blockers we were taking listed low platelet levels as one possible side effect."

Their doctor didn't believe them at first. "I was just a kid, and here I was presenting evidence about our drugs to our doctor. He kind of blew me off at first." But once she presented her research, the doctor agreed to take Kim's sister off the drug for a trial period.

"It felt good to teach him something," she told me. "And after that first conversation, he was really open. Honestly, that experience was one of the things that cemented my desire to go to medical school."

We like to think that our doctors always have all the relevant information about our prescriptions, our conditions, and our treatments. But that's simply not the case. Our body of medical knowledge is too vast for any one person to absorb, let alone comprehend. That's why there are so many specialties within the field; some of us want to stay broad, while others want to go deep. And no matter our field, keeping up with the latest advancements can be a full-time venture in and of itself.

When you use the vast resources available online to do your own research, you may end up discovering something that even your doctor doesn't know. This doesn't mean that the doctor is not good, just that the information hasn't come across his or her radar yet. I know many PCPs and specialists who love when their patients come in with research. Why? Because patients are looking for information specific to their condition or combination of conditions, which means their searches are deep and targeted, not broad and general.

That said, there is a lot of quackery out there in the digital world, so it's important to vet your information sources carefully before drawing any conclusions. Stick to reputable patient education sites like those created by WebMD, the Cleveland Clinic, the Mayo Clinic, the National Institutes of Health, the Centers for Disease Control and Prevention, Drugs.com, and of course the

Sex and Gender Women's Health Collaborative—as well as, if you find them interesting, peer-reviewed literature and scientific journals on sites like PubMed.

If alternative health and medicine is your thing, it may be harder to find vetted information, especially in the United States; however, a growing number of European, Chinese, and Japanese research teams are investigating acupuncture, energy healing, aromatherapy, and other "alternative" modalities and publishing their findings in international journals. (PubMed also includes international publications, so start there.)

Here are some ways that you can use the internet to your advantage when it comes to your health and well-being:

- Research your current conditions and make a list of possible treatments, meds, and tests to discuss with your doctor, especially if you feel like you aren't getting the relief you need from your current regimen.

- Research your current prescriptions, especially around sex differences and interactions with other prescriptions. For example, if you're on warfarin, Lipitor, and birth control, a simple Google search of "warfarin and Lipitor" will turn up dozens of articles about the ways in which these drugs have been observed to interact. Another search for "Lipitor and birth control" will offer more information about that interaction. Remember, medications aren't necessarily studied in combination, even when those combinations are common across millions of people.

It's also important to note that the combination of online research sessions and the known tendency of our system to minimize women's pain can result in you, as a woman, feeling even less seen and cared for, especially if you don't share with your providers what you have discovered and what you fear may be happening in your body. After all, almost every symptom described on WebMD or other sites has a few dire causes attached to it, and it can often be unclear whether these scenarios should be of real concern to you.

For example, if a woman comes into my ED with intense abdominal pain, I immediately start looking for things like ovarian cysts, appendicitis, or small bowel obstruction. However, if she has a family history of uterine cancer (and Google has verified that her symptoms may be consistent with that), those things may be the least of her concerns. If I as a provider don't address her cancer fear because I don't have a record of this family history, she may feel slighted, even though I did my job to the best of my ability in the moment. She didn't just come to the ED because of her pain; she came to verify that her pain wasn't caused by a tumor.

The lesson here: don't be afraid to speak to your providers about what you've discovered online. You're not undermining their work by doing your own research. In fact, what you've learned may actually empower you to have a better and more detailed conversation—and, if you fear something may be really wrong, to get the information you need to either allay that fear or get an actual diagnosis.

Here are some ways you can translate your online research into conversations with your providers:

- Save, print, or take a screenshot of the website where you found your information or areas of concern. That way, your doctor knows exactly what you are referencing.

- Take notes (on paper or your phone) about what aspects of your symptoms are causing you concern. You can reference this in your conversation so you don't forget to bring up vital details.

Advocacy

As I've stressed throughout this book, the most important way you can contribute to creating change in medicine is to make your voice heard. I've given you some tools to do that on an individual level in your conversations with your providers; however, you may be inspired to do more. In this section, we'll discuss some ways that you can participate in advocacy.

The first and most obvious way, of course, is to donate to research and advocacy foundations and agencies. Look for reputable, national agencies whose values align with your own. The British Heart Foundation, Cancer Research U.K. and The Stroke Association are well-known examples, but there are also many smaller organizations (such as the Sex and Gender Women's Health Collaborative) that are doing a great job of raising awareness and funding research.

You can also support research in sex and gender medicine more directly by contributing to specific divisions within your local universities and training hospitals. You could specify that you want to support a specific research project, fund the training of a new fellow, or support direct patient services on a local level through groups like the Patient Advocate Foundation.

While many people do opt to donate, financial contributions are only one way to support change in the medical field. Alone or with a group of like-minded individuals, you can do your part to help spread the word about how and why sex matters in medicine.

Here are some ideas for advocacy that don't cost anything but can be hugely effective:

- Join a medical research trial. If we want to learn more about how our current drugs, treatments, and protocols affect women, we need women to participate in the research process. Many trials even offer reimbursement for travel and expenses.
- Join a support group (or create your own). Knowing you're not alone and having people with whom to converse about your condition and/or medical experience is invaluable. You can also delegate research tasks among the group, share experiences about your interactions with providers and hospitals, and connect with researchers working in your field.
- Write to your local paper or to relevant online publications. Sharing your experience, your questions, and your insights not only helps other patients but also helps practitioners and facilities see where they need to be putting their focus to continually improve.
- Harness the power of social media to share your story, meet others who have had similar experiences, and connect with like-minded people around the globe.
- Meet with hospital management to address any concerns you have and share your experience. Most hospitals have media liaisons or public relations staff who are responsible for creating the "public face" of the hospital; they are a good place to start if you have a complaint or feel like you aren't being heard.

However you choose to do so, always remember that it's important for you as a woman to make your voice heard in the medical world. Remember, your participation, your donation, or your story could be the key that makes it possible for others to get the treatment they need.

What Matters—Your Key Takeaways

- A key determinant of outcomes is the level of trust patients have in their provider. It's important to cultivate relationships with your PCP and other core providers that empower you to have authentic conversations and share all your questions and concerns freely.
- Always ask your providers about sex- and gender-specific tests, procedures, prescriptions, and dosing. This will open a conversation about the health pathways that are best suited to your unique biology.
- Planning ahead can help you create the best possible outcomes in your provider visits, hospital stays, and other medical interactions. Simple things like saving your medical information to your phone, creating paper or digital lists of medications and dosages, and designating an informed and competent advocate can make a huge difference and ensure you get the highest possible quality of care.
- Do your research online—but do it in a way that gets you the best possible information. Share this information freely with your providers. Who knows—you might even teach them something!
- Above all, be your own advocate. No one's voice should take precedence over yours when it comes to your body and your health care.

AFTERWORD

A FEW MONTHS AGO, my mom was shopping at the mall with my father when she started having pronounced symptoms including shortness of breath, chest discomfort, and fatigue. My dad rushed to the nearest security guard, who in turn called the mall's emergency medical technician (EMT).

When the EMT arrived, he asked my mom a flurry of questions. "Does it feel like your chest is being crushed? Is the pain radiating down your left arm?"

My mom, feisty as ever despite her fear, narrowed her eyes at him and announced, "That's *not* how women have heart attacks!"

"So how do women have heart attacks?" the EMT asked, obviously taken aback.

Mom proceeded to educate him.

By the time they finished this conversation, the EMT was convinced that my mom had the right of it—and my mom was feeling better. Rather than going to the hospital, she contacted her primary care provider, who was able to see her later that day.

Before he left, Mom made the EMT promise to research sex differences in emergency medicine so that he wouldn't misidentify any other female cardiac events. He agreed.

Thankfully, my mom is fine—and I'm proud of her for the role she played in her own care. Like her, I attribute her quick recovery in part to the fact that no time was wasted in her diagnosis. She knew the symptoms and signs of a female-pattern heart attack and was able to communicate clearly and precisely with her providers as a result.

This story is a perfect example of how women patients, armed with knowledge about how their sex makes them unique, can change the way they receive care in our current medical system, right now. You too can put what you've learned in this book to use in real-world situations—whether on behalf of yourself or someone you love.

As I've shared, change within our medical system *is* happening. It's slow, but now that we've gotten the ball rolling, it's also inevitable. We can't go back to where we were before; we can't unlearn what we have learned.

My wish for you, reader, is that you don't lose faith in medicine as we work to perpetuate change. Science is remarkable; it's also fallible and evolutionary. Those of us who work with human biology on a daily basis are constantly pushing toward a new level of understanding, clarity, and excellence.

I'm honored and thrilled to be at the forefront of sex and gender medicine in this exciting time. We are learning more than ever before, and all the research, education, and discussion that has happened over the last ten-plus years has finally started to bear fruit. I know that my colleagues are just as excited as I am—even though we still have a long way to go if we want to get to a place where women's bodies are as well respected, well studied, and well treated as men's. We have a lot to learn and a lot to unlearn, but we are willing, open, and excited about the impact of the changes to come on our health as individuals and as a society.

Revolution may start with one person or a small, select group of visionaries—but it never ends that way. Each of us has the power to harness our "a-ha" moments, our knowledge of our own bodies, and our professional expertise to create a cascade of change in the medical world.

I can't do this alone. But I know that once women understand the power they have to effect positive and lasting change in their own health and the health of other women, I won't have to. We will move forward, together, one step at a time.

Yours in health,
Dr. Alyson J. McGregor

ACKNOWLEDGMENTS

So many people have contributed to the development of this book. I am grateful for them all.

To my agent, Andrew Stuart, who reached out to me with the idea to write a book years ago: thank you for being patient enough to stick with me until I was ready.

To Bruce Becker, MD, with whom I conceived the original idea for this book: thank you for helping me realize the value of telling my story as well as sharing the facts.

To the publishing team at Hachette Books/Hachette Go, especially my editor, Renee: you have approached this project with the same enthusiasm as I have. Thank you for supporting this message and ensuring its outreach.

To my writing partner, Bryna Haynes, without whom this book would never have happened: thank you for being all in—not just for me but for the message that needed to be heard and understood across the globe. You were so generous with your guidance and expertise, your lightness and laughter. You made writing this book an enjoyable experience!

To the colleagues and beta readers who contributed their valuable time and energy to read, comment, and gently point out where I didn't know what I didn't know, Resa E. Lewiss, MD; Esther K. Choo, MD, MPH; Sheryl L. Heron, MD, MPH, FACEP; Laleh Gharahbaghian, MD, FACEP, FAAEM; and Taneisha Wilson, MD: I am grateful for the power of our collective intelligence.

To the doctors who contributed their knowledge to expand our discussion, Barbara Roberts, MD; Basmah Safdar, MD, FACEP; Sharonne Hayes, MD; Paula J. Rackoff, MD; Lindsey J. Gurin, MD; and C. Noel Bairey Merz, MD: thank you for sharing your wisdom with me and with everyone who will read this work.

To all my colleagues who share this journey with me, particularly Marjorie R. Jenkins, MD, FACP: thank you for helping to reshape our understanding of women's bodies in a collaborative, collective way on a national and international stage. I have learned from you in endless ways.

To the courageous colleagues working in this field, faculty members, residents, medical students, undergraduate students, committee members, and organization leaders: thank you for all that you have done and continue to do to shift and redefine the status quo. Equality is imperative; it translates to improved health for all.

To the faculty and leaders at the Warren Alpert Medical School of Brown University (my academic home since completing my medical training) and the Department of Emergency Medicine: thank you for allowing me to pursue an avenue of study that was previously uncharted. This support to establish the first Division of

Acknowledgments

Sex and Gender in Emergency Medicine gave me a framework for research, education, and advocacy.

To my friends, near and far: thank you for seeing me, hearing me, and loving me. Every good revolutionary needs a sounding board, and for me, that person is Erin Sarris. We met in nursery school and became instant BFFs. You have always been the person I turn to when I need to talk life, politics, and feminist theory. Thanks also to Kerri Ialongo and Julez Weinberg for listening to me on my sex and gender soapbox at every get-together, cocktail party, dinner, wedding, funeral, graduation, and holiday; you always offer sage advice and compassionate support.

To my family, without whom I would never have come this far: my deepest love and gratitude to you. To my mother, Joanne, and father, Peter: love and support are your currency—and I won the lottery. Thanks for reminding me that I can do anything in this world and for giving me the tools to succeed. To Robyn and Scott: you are the best family cheerleaders ever. You're there for me no matter what. To my in-laws, Nancy and Jerry, thank you for your wonderful support and caring.

And finally, to my husband, Eric, whose insight and love lift me up in so many ways: thank you for sharing this journey with me. Since we were fresh out of college, both studying hard to get into med school, then learning emergency medicine together, then exploring how the system could be made better, you've always encouraged me to go for it—to be the advocate, to pursue my mission, to be the voice for those who need to be heard. I love you (and our dogs Olive, Feta, and Basil) always.

YOUR PERSONAL MEDICAL RECONCILIATION (MED REC)

Write all your pertinent medical information in the space below. Copy or tear out these pages and carry them with you to all medical encounters. Alternately, download a PDF version at: www.alysonmcgregor.com/personal-med-rec.

My Name _____

My Birth/Biological Sex _____

My Current Sex/Gender Identity_____

My Current Primary Care Physician

    Name _____

    Address _____

    Phone _____

    Email _____

Your Personal Medical Reconciliation (Med Rec)

My Current Specialists and Nonprimary Care Providers

(add as many as needed):

Name _____

Address _____

Phone _____

Email _____

Date of my last period _____

My typical menstrual/premenstrual symptoms are:

My Current Contraception Regimen

Include all forms of contraception, including pills, implants, IUDs, condoms, etc.

My Current Medical Conditions/Diagnoses

My Surgical History

My Recent Doctor's Visits

Include primary care physician, specialists, emergency departments, urgent care centers, etc.

My Recent Tests/Imaging and Their Results

Include X-rays, CT scans, ultrasounds, EKGs, MRIs, stress tests, etc.

My Current and Past Pharmaceuticals

Include even those prescriptions you don't take on a regular basis.

Medication Name	Generic? Y/N	Dose (in mg/mcg)	Frequency (times per day)	Notes

My Current Over-the-Counter Medications

Include pain relievers, allergy and cold medicines, herbal supplements, vitamins, CBD products, etc.

Supplement/Med Name	Dose (in mg/mcg)	Frequency (times per day)	Notes

My Allergies

Include foods, medications, and other substances.

Allergy	Typical Reaction to This Allergen

My Current Conditions

Include all current disease diagnoses (e.g., diabetes, microvascular disease), mental health–related diagnoses (e.g., anxiety, depression), pain conditions, etc. Then describe as accurately as possible how the symptoms of that condition usually feel in your body and mind.

Condition	The typical symptoms I associate with this condition

My Drug and Alcohol Use

Include alcohol (wine, beer, liquor), marijuana, and any other recreational substances.

Substance	How many times (per day/week/month)

I am a habitual smoker   ☐ Y   ☐ N

I am a social smoker   ☐ Y   ☐ N

    Number of cigarettes per day/week? _____

I use a vaping system   ☐ Y   ☐ N

    If so, how often? _____

My vaping use includes: THC?   ☐ Y   ☐ N

                                    CBD?   ☐ Y   ☐ N

                                  Nicotine?   ☐ Y   ☐ N

appendix b

QUICK REFERENCE QUESTIONS

Tear out these pages to bring with you to your providers' offices as an aid to your conversations. Or download and print the complete list at www.alysonmcgregor.com/questions-list.

For a more complete list and associated discussion, revisit Chapter 10.

Questions to ask your primary care provider (PCP):

- "What are the latest recommendations for women of my age around…?"
  - Yearly screenings and blood work
  - Breast exams (including mammography)
  - Colonoscopy
  - Pap tests
  - Other routine testing
- "How often do I need to do the above exams, and why?"

- "Do you perform Pap tests, pelvic exams, and breast exams, or do I need to see my OB/GYN for that?" (Not all PCPs provide these services.)
- "Are you aware of the latest research on sex and gender in your field?"
- "Do you observe that your female patients and patients of color have equal outcomes to your male patients?"

Questions to ask your PCP about specific medical issues:

- "What is my medical condition?" (Feel free to say, "Can you explain this to me in nonmedical terms so I can understand it better?")
- "Please tell me what I can expect with this prescription/these prescriptions. Are there any side effects I need to watch for? Is this the right dose for me based on my sex, age, weight, and health conditions?"

Questions to ask your specialist(s):

- "Have you studied sex differences in your discipline?"
- "Does this test/procedure you're recommending take into account my personal biology?"
- "Have you noticed any disparity in outcomes between your male and female patients?"
- "What are the alternatives if this test doesn't give us the answers we're looking for?"
- "Are there side effects of this test/procedure that I should be aware of as a woman?"
- "Will this test/procedure be influenced or impacted by my birth control/pregnancy/breastfeeding/HRT?"

Questions for your PCP and/or prescribing specialist(s) about pharmaceuticals

- "Are the meds I am taking the right ones for my sex, race/ethnicity, and stage of life?"
- "Am I taking sex-appropriate doses, or do we need to adjust my prescriptions?"
- "Is this medication tested in women? If so, are there different dosing guidelines I should be aware of?"
- "Will this prescription affect my birth control or HRT?"
- "Is this medication a generic, and if so, how might that affect me? Has this generic been studied in women?"
- "Does this medication prolong the QT interval? How might this affect me given my other medications?"
- "I've observed that I feel different since I started this new generic, and I'm concerned it may not be metabolizing as well as my former medication. Is there another affordable brand I could switch to?"

Questions to ask if you are prescribed pain medication:

- "Is this considered an opiate?"
- "Should I take it only if I have pain?"
- "Can you give me a list of alternatives to opiates and other potentially addictive medications?"

Questions to ask as a woman of color:

Of individual doctors and specialists
- "Do you feel that women of color have the same outcomes as white patients in your practice?"

- "Do you see many women of color in your practice?"
- "Are you willing to hear and discuss my concerns about racial and cultural bias in medical practice?"
- "Are you willing to accommodate [my personal, cultural, or religious concerns] in the course of visits and treatments?"

Of hospitals, urgent care centers, and medical groups
- "Have your doctors and staff received education in cultural competence?"
- "What is your current level of diversity among doctors and staff?"
- "Do you have experience with [individual cultural/religious practices]? Will you be willing to accommodate my particular requests and concerns?"

RESOURCES

Books

- Boston Women's Health Book Collective. *Our Bodies, Ourselves.* Rev. ed. New York: Atria Books, 2011.
- Dusenbery, Maya. *Doing Harm: The Truth About How Bad Medicine and Lazy Science Leave Women Dismissed, Misdiagnosed, and Sick.* New York: HarperOne, 2018.
- Dwass, Emily. *Diagnosis Female: How Medical Bias Endangers Women's Health.* Lanham, MD: Rowman & Littlefield, 2019.
- Glezerman, Marek. *Gender Medicine: The Groundbreaking New Science of Gender- and Sex-Related Diagnosis and Treatment.* New York: Harry N. Abrams, 2016.
- Killermann, Sam. *A Guide to Gender: The Social Justice Advocate's Handbook.* 2nd ed. Austin, TX: Impetus Books, 2017.
- Legato, Marianne, ed. *Principles of Gender-Specific Medicine.* 3rd ed. Cambridge, MA: Academic Press, 2017.
- Mark, Saralyn. *Stellar Medicine: A Journey Through the Universe of Women's Health.* New York: Brick Tower Press, 2012.
- McGregor, Alyson J., Esther K. Choo, and Bruce M. Becker. *Sex and Gender in Acute Care Medicine.* New York: Cambridge University Press, 2016. doi:10.1017/CBO9781107705944.

- Perez, Caroline Criado. *Invisible Women: Data Bias in a World Designed for Men.* New York: Abrams Press, 2019.
- Schenck-Gustafsson, K., P. R. DeCola, D. W. Pfaff, and D. S. Pisetsky. *Handbook of Clinical Gender Medicine.* Berlin: Karger Publishers, 2012.

Online Research Resources

- British Heart Foundation: https://www.bhf.org.uk/information support/heart-matters-magazine/medical/women
- British Medical Association: https://www.bma.org.uk/events/2019/november/overcoming-gender-bias-in-medicine
- British Medical Journal: https://www.bmj.com/content/363/bmj.k424
- Canadian Institutes of Health Research–Institute of Gender and Health: http://www.cihr-irsc.gc.ca/e/8673.html
- Embryo Project Encyclopaedia: https://embryo.asu.edu/pages/studies-thalidomides-effects-rodent-embryos-1962-2008
- Endometriosis: https://endometriosis-uk.org/news/it-takes-average-75-years-get-diagnosis-endometriosis-it-shouldnt-37491#.XmEeH6hKhPY
- Facility for Sexual and Reproductive Healthcare, "FSRH CEU Guidance: Drug Interactions with Hormonal Contraception (January 2017, last reviewed 2019)": https://www.fsrh.org/standards-and-guidance/documents/ceu-clinical-guidance-drug-interactions-with-hormonal
- Food and Drug Administration, "Drug Trials Snapshots": https://www.fda.gov/drugs/drug-approvals-and-databases/drug-trials-snapshots
- LGBT: https://lgbt.foundation/pride-in-practice
- Mental Health First Aid: https://mhfaengland.org/mhfa-centre/research-and-evaluation/mental-health-statistics/
- National Centre for Biotechnology Information: https://www.ncbi.nlm.nih.gov/pubmed/12690218
- NHS: https://www.nhs.uk/news/mental-health/women-are-more-likely-to-suffer-from-anxiety-than-men/

- PubMed, an online resource from the National Institutes of Health and National Libraries of Medicine providing millions of medical journal articles: https://www.ncbi.nlm.nih.gov/pubmed
- Society for Women's Health Research: https://swhr.org
- Stroke Association: https://www.stroke.org.uk/sites/default/files/state_of_the_nation_2017_final_1.pdf
- Women's Health Research at Yale University: https://medicine.yale.edu/whr
- Yellow Card Scheme: https://yellowcard.mhra.gov.uk/

Institutes/Organizations

- American Medical Women's Association, Sex and Gender Health Collaborative: https://www.amwa-doc.org/sghc
- Cedars-Sinai Hospital, Barbra Streisand Women's Heart Center: https://www.cedars-sinai.org/programs/heart/clinical/womens-heart.html
- Centre de Recherche de l'Institut Universitaire de Gériatrie de Montréal, Cara Tannenbaum profile and deprescribing brochures: http://www.criugm.qc.ca/en/researchers/laboratory-directors/63-cara-tannenbaum.html
- European Society of Gender Health Medicine: http://www.gendermedicine.org
- Food and Drug Administration, Office of Women's Health: https://www.fda.gov/about-fda/office-commissioner/office-womens-health
- Foundation for Gender-Specific Medicine: https://gendermed.org
- Gendered Innovations at Stanford University: https://genderedinnovations.stanford.edu
- Impact of Gender/Sex on Innovation and Novel Technologies: https://www.igiant.org
- International Society of Gender Medicine: http://www.isogem.eu
- Karolinska Institute, Stockholm, Sweden: https://ki.se/en/research/about-cfg
- Laura Bush Institute for Women's Health: https://www.sexandgenderhealth.org

- Office of Research on Women's Health, National Institutes of Health: https://orwh.od.nih.gov
- Organization for the Study of Sex Differences: https://www.ossdweb.org

Telemedicine and Remote Services

- CVS Health virtual care offerings: https://cvshealth.com/newsroom/press-releases/cvs-healths-minuteclinic-introduces-new-virtual-care-offering
- JeffConnect at Jefferson University: https://hospitals.jefferson.edu/jeffconnect/jeffconnect-telehealth-consulting.html

Apps

- Google medical ID app: https://play.google.com/store/apps/details?id=app.medicalid.free&hl=en_US
- MediSafe app for tracking medications: https://www.medisafeapp.com
- Meds Agenda to organize meds and doses: https://apps.apple.com/us/app/meds-agenda/id520098571

Films

- *Ms. Diagnosed: The Movie*: https://www.msdiagnosedfilm.com

NOTES

Chapter 1

1. A. H. E. M. Maas and Y. E. A. Appelman, "Gender Differences in Coronary Heart Disease," *Netherlands Heart Journal* 18, no. 12 (2010): 598–602, https://www.ncbi.nlm.nih.gov/pmc/articles/PMC3018605.

2. Steven R. Messé et al., "Why Are Acute Ischemic Stroke Patients Not Receiving IV tPA? Results from a National Registry," *Neurology* 87, no. 15 (2016): 1565–1574. doi: 10.1212/WNL.0000000000003198; American Academy of Neurology (AAN), "Women, Minorities May Be Undertreated for Stroke," *ScienceDaily*, https://www.sciencedaily.com/releases/2016/09/160914172413.htm.

3. Romy Ubrich et al., "Sex Differences in Long-Term Mortality Among Acute Myocardial Infarction Patients: Results from the ISAR-RISK and ART Studies," *PLOS ONE* 12, no. 10 (2017): e0186783. doi: 10.1371/journal.pone.0186783; Technical University of Munich (TUM), "Women More Likely to Die in the First Year After a Heart Attack," *ScienceDaily*, https://www.sciencedaily.com/releases/2017/10/171025105045.htm.

Chapter 2

1. Katherine A. Liu and Natalie A. Dipietro Mager, "Women's Involvement in Clinical Trials: Historical Perspective and Future Implications," *Pharmacy Practice* (Granada) 14, no. 1 (2016): 708. doi: 10.18549/PharmPract.2016.01.708.

2. M. S. Arruda et al., "Time Elapsed from Onset of Symptoms to Diagnosis of Endometriosis in a Cohort Study of Brazilian Women," *Human Reproduction* 18, no. 4 (2003): 756–759. doi: 10.1093/HumRep/deg136; G. K. Husby, R. S. Haugen, and M. H. Moen, "Diagnostic Delay in Women with Pain and Endometriosis," *Acta Obstetricia et Gynecologica Scandinavica* 82, no. 7 (2003): 649–653, https://www.ncbi.nlm.nih.gov/pubmed/12790847.

3. Janet Woodcock, MD, John Whyte, MD, MPH, and Milena Lolic, MD, MS, "2017 Drug Trials Snapshot Summary Report," U.S. Food and Drug Administration, January 2017, https://www.fda.gov/media/112373/download.

4. Natalie Jacewicz, "Why Are Health Studies So White?," *The Atlantic*, June 16, 2016, https://www.theatlantic.com/health/archive/2016/06/why-are-health-studies-so-white/487046.

5. Steven R. Messé et al., "Why Are Acute Ischemic Stroke Patients Not Receiving IV tPA? Results from a National Registry," *Neurology* 87, no. 15 (2016): 1565–1574. doi: 10.1212/WNL.0000000000003198; American Academy of Neurology (AAN), "Women, Minorities May Be Undertreated for Stroke," *ScienceDaily*, https://www.sciencedaily.com/releases/2016/09/160914172413.htm.

6. C. R. Bankhead et al., "Identifying Symptoms of Ovarian Cancer: A Qualitative and Quantitative Study," *BJOG* 115, no. 8 (2008): 1008–1014. doi: 10.1111/j.1471-0528.2008.01772.x.

7. Ronald Wyatt, MD, MHA, "Pain and Ethnicity," *AMA Journal of Ethics* 15, no. 5 (2013): 449–454. doi: 10.1001/virtualmentor.2013.15.5.pfor1-1305.

Chapter 3

1. Thomas Emil Christensen et al., "Neuroticism, Depression and Anxiety in Takotsubo Cardiomyopathy," *BMC Cardiovascular Disorders* 16 (2016): 118. doi: 10.1186/s12872-016-0277-4.

2. Oras A. Alabas et al., "Sex Differences in Treatments, Relative Survival, and Excess Mortality Following Acute Myocardial Infarction: National Cohort Study Using the SWEDEHEART Registry," *Journal of the American Heart Association* 6, no. 12 (2017). doi: 10.1161/JAHA.117.007123.

3. "Women and Heart Disease," Centers for Disease Control and Prevention, page last reviewed May 2019, https://www.cdc.gov/heartdisease/women.htm.

4. Randy Young, "The Way to Women's Heart Health," Cardiovascular Business.com, January 7, 2019, https://www.cardiovascularbusiness.com/topics/structural-congenital-heart-disease/way-womens-heart-health.

5. "AHA Guidelines Recognize Preeclampsia as CVD Risk Factor," Preeclampsia.org, last updated February 2014, https://www.preeclampsia.org/the-news/53-health-information/517-aha-guidelines-recognize-preeclampsia-as-cvd-risk-factor; Cheryl Bushnell, MD, MHS, FAHA et al., "Guidelines for the Prevention of Stroke in Women: A Statement for Healthcare Professionals from the American Heart Association/American Stroke Association," *Stroke* 45, no. 5 (2014): 1545–1588. doi: 10.1161/01.str.0000442009.06663.48.

6. "The Cardiac Risks of Rheumatoid Arthritis," Cleveland HeartLab. August 7, 2017, http://www.clevelandheartlab.com/blog/the-cardiac-risks-of-rheumatoid-arthritis.

7. Deborah P. M. Symmons and Sherine E. Gabriel, "Epidemiology of CVD in Rheumatic Disease, with a Focus on RA and SLE," *Nature Reviews Rheumatology* 7 (2011): 399–408, https://www.nature.com/articles/nrrheum.2011.75.

8. Una McCann, MD, "Anxiety and Heart Disease," Johns Hopkins Medicine, https://www.hopkinsmedicine.org/heart_vascular_institute/clinical_services/centers_excellence/womens_cardiovascular_health_center/patient_information/health_topics/anxiety_heart_disease.html.

9. Olivia Remes, Carol Brayne, Rianne van der Linde, and Louise Lafortune, "A Systematic Review of Reviews on the Prevalence of Anxiety Disorders in Adult Populations," *Brain and Behavior* 6, no. 7 (2016), e00497, doi: 10.1002/brb3.497.

10. "The Link Between Anxiety and Heart Disease," Magnolia Regional Health Center, December 18, 2017, https://www.mrhc.org/blog/heart-disease/the-link-between-anxiety-heart-disease.

11. "New Study: Women More Likely to Die After a Heart Attack Due to Unequal Treatment," World Heart Federation, January 10, 2018, https://www.world-heart-federation.org/news/new-study-women-likely-die-heart-attack-due-unequal-treatment; Oras A. Alabas et al., "Sex Differences in Treatments, Relative Survival, and Excess Mortality Following Acute

Myocardial Infarction: National Cohort Study Using the SWEDEHEART Registry," *Journal of the American Heart Association* 6, no. 12 (2017). doi: 10.1161/JAHA.117.007123.

12. P. Dewan, "Differential Impact of Heart Failure with Reduced Ejection Fraction on Men and Women," *Journal of the American College of Cardiology* 73, no. 1 (2019): 29–40. doi: 10.1016/j.jacc.2018.09.081.

13. Jason Kashdan, "Healthy Heart May Help Men Battle Cancer, Study Finds," *CBS News*, March 27, 2015, https://www.cbsnews.com/news/cancer-study -men-finds-cardio-exercise-may-reduce-risk-cancer-death-risk. Dr. David Agus is the commentator. Mention happens at 1:00 with a question from the anchor.

14. Laura F. DeFina et al., "Association of All-Cause and Cardiovascular Mortality with High Levels of Physical Activity and Concurrent Coronary Artery Calcification," *JAMA Cardiology* 4, no. 2 (2019):174–181. doi:10.1001/jamacardio.2018.4628.

15. Gretchen Reynolds, "Can You Get Too Much Exercise? What the Heart Tells Us," *New York Times*, February 6, 2019, https://www.nytimes.com /2019/02/06/well/move/can-you-get-too-much-exercise-what-the -heart-tells-us.html.

16. A. M. Napoli, E. K. Choo, and A. McGregor, "Gender Disparities in Stress Test Utilization in Chest Pain Unit Patients Based upon the Ordering Physician's Gender," *Critical Pathways in Cardiology* 13, no. 4 (2014):152– 155. doi: 10.1097/HPC.0000000000000026.

17. Napoli, Choo, and McGregor, "Gender Disparities in Stress Test Utilization."

18. Randy Young, "The Way to Women's Heart Health," Cardiovascular Business.com, January 7, 2019, https://www.cardiovascularbusiness.com /topics/structural-congenital-heart-disease/way-womens-heart-health; L. S. Mehta et al., "Acute Myocardial Infarction in Women: A Scientific Statement from the American Heart Association," *Circulation* 133, no. 9 (2016): 916–947. doi: 10.1161/CIR.0000000000000351.

19. Hypothermia After Cardiac Arrest Study Group, "Mild Therapeutic Hypothermia to Improve the Neurologic Outcome After Cardiac Arrest," *New England Journal of Medicine* 346 (2002): 549–556. doi: 10.1056/NEJM oa012689.

20. Jessica E. Morse et al., "Evidence-Based Pregnancy Testing in Clinical Trials: Recommendations from a Multi-Stakeholder Development Process," *PLOS ONE* 13, no. 9 (2018): e0202474. doi: 10.1371/journal.pone.0202474.

21. Meytal Avgil Tsadok, PhD, et al., "Sex Differences in Dabigatran Use, Safety, and Effectiveness in a Population-Based Cohort of Patients with Atrial Fibrillation," *Circulation: Cardiovascular Quality and Outcomes* 8 (2015): 593–599. doi: 10.1161/CIRCOUTCOMES.114.001398.

22. "Women and Stroke," CDC.gov, https://www.cdc.gov/stroke/docs/women_stroke_factsheet.pdf.

23. "Women and Stroke."

24. Caroline Cassels, "ISC 2009: Women with Stroke, TIA, More Likely Than Men to Report Mental Status Change," *Medscape*, February 24, 2009, https://www.medscape.com/viewarticle/588640.

25. T. E. Madsen et al., "Analysis of Tissue Plasminogen Activator Eligibility by Sex in the Greater Cincinnati/Northern Kentucky Stroke Study," *Stroke* 46, no. 3 (2015): 717–721. doi: 10.1161/STROKEAHA.114.006737.

26. Mathew Reeves, PhD, et al., "Sex Differences in the Use of Intravenous rt-PA Thrombolysis Treatment for Acute Ischemic Stroke: A Meta-Analysis," *Stroke* 40 (2009): 1743–1749, https://www.ahajournals.org/doi/pdf/10.1161/STROKEAHA.108.543181.

Chapter 4

1. M. Manteuffel et al., "Influence of Patient Sex and Gender on Medication Use, Adherence, and Prescribing Alignment with Guidelines," *Journal of Women's Health* 23, no. 2 (2014): 112–199. doi: 10.1089/jwh.2012.3972.

2. Giselle Sarganas, "Epidemiology of Symptomatic Drug-Induced Long QT Syndrome and Torsade de Pointes in Germany," *EP Europace* 16, no. 1 (2014): 101–108. doi: 10.1093/europace/eut214.

3. Teresa Chu, PhD, "Gender Differences in Pharmacokinetics in Pharmacology," *U.S. Pharmacist* 39, no. 9 (2014): 40–43.

4. "Absorption Rate Factors," University of Notre Dame, https://mcwell.nd.edu/your-well-being/physical-well-being/alcohol/absorption-rate-factors.

5. "GAO-01-286R Drug Safety: Most Drugs Withdrawn in Recent Years Had Greater Health Risks for Women," GAO.gov, https://www.gao.gov/assets/100/90642.pdf.

6. Jo Jones et al., "Current Contraceptive Use in the United States, 2006–2010, and Changes in Patterns of Use Since 1995," *National Health Statistics Reports* 60 (2012), https://www.cdc.gov/nchs/data/nhsr/nhsr060.pdf.

7. David J. Waxman and Minita G. Holloway, "Sex Differences in the Expression of Hepatic Drug Metabolizing Enzymes," *Molecular Pharmacology* 76 (2009): 215–228, https://www.ncbi.nlm.nih.gov/pubmed/19483103.

8. Francis Collins, "We Need Better Drugs—Now," TED, April 2012, https://www.ted.com/talks/francis_collins_we_need_better_drugs_now.

9. "FDA Adverse Event Reporting System (FAERS) Public Dashboard," FDA.gov, https://www.fda.gov/drugs/guidancecomplianceregulatoryinformation/surveillance/adversedrugeffects/ucm070093.htm.

10. Paul M. Ridker, "The JUPITER Trial: Results, Controversies, and Implications for Prevention," *Circulation: Cardiovascular Quality and Outcomes* 2 (2009): 279–285. doi: 10.1161/CIRCOUTCOMES.109.868299.

11. Pamela E. Scott et al., "Participation of Women in Clinical Trials Supporting FDA Approval of Cardiovascular Drugs," *Journal of the American College of Cardiology* 71, no. 18 (2018). doi: 10.1016/j.jacc.2018.02.070.

12. "Lisinopril—Drug Summary," PDR.net, https://www.pdr.net/drug-summary/Prinivil-lisinopril-376.

13. D. M. Rabi, MD MSc, et al., "Reporting on Sex-Based Analysis in Clinical Trials of Angiotensin-Converting Enzyme Inhibitor and Angiotensin Receptor Blocker Efficacy," *Canadian Journal of Cardiology* 24, no. 6 (2008): 491–496. https://www.ncbi.nlm.nih.gov/pmc/articles/PMC2643194.

14. Helen M. Pettinati, PhD, et al., "Gender Differences with High Dose Naltrexone in Cocaine and Alcohol Dependent Patients," *Journal of Substance Abuse Treatment* 34, no. 4 (2008): 378–390. doi: 10.1016/j.jsat.2007.05.011.

15. M.-L. Chen et al., "Pharmacokinetic Analysis of Bioequivalence Trials: Implications for Sex-Related Issues in Clinical Pharmacology and Biopharmaceutics," *Clinical Pharmacology & Therapeutics* 68, no. 5 (2000): 510–521. doi: 10.1067/mcp.2000.111184.

16. G. Koren, H. Nordeng, and S. MacLeod, "Gender Differences in Drug Bioequivalence: Time to Rethink Practices," *Clinical Pharmacology & Therapeutics* 93, no. 3 (2013): 260–262. doi: 10.1038/clpt.2012.233.

Chapter 5

1. Gunilla Risberg, Eva E. Johansson, and Katarina Hamberg, "A Theoretical Model for Analysing Gender Bias in Medicine," *International Journal for Equity in Health* 8, no. 28 (2009). doi:10.1186/1475-9276-8-28.

2. B. G. Kane et al., "Gender Differences in CDC Guideline Compliance for STIs in Emergency Departments," *Western Journal of Emergency Medicine* 18, no. 3 (2017): 390–397. doi: 10.5811/westjem.2016.12.32440.

3. David Gomez, MD, PhD, et al., "Gender-Associated Differences in Access to Trauma Center Care: A Population-Based Analysis," *Surgery* 152, no. 2 (2012): 179–185. doi: https://doi.org/10.1016/j.surg.2012.04.006.

4. A. Gupta et al., "Gender Disparity and the Appropriateness of Myocardial Perfusion Imaging," *Journal of Nuclear Cardiology* 18, no. 4 (2011): 588–594. doi: 10.1007/s12350-011-9368-x; A. M. Chang et al., "Gender Bias in Cardiovascular Testing Persists After Adjustment for Presenting Characteristics and Cardiac Risk," *Academic Emergency Medicine* 14, no. 7 (2007): 599–605. doi: 10.1197/j.aem.2007.03.1355.

5. J. H. Pope et al., "Missed Diagnoses of Acute Cardiac Ischemia in the Emergency Department," *New England Journal of Medicine* 342, no. 16 (2000): 1163–1170. doi: 10.1056/NEJM200004203421603.

6. Rohit Verma, Yatan Pal Singh Balhara, and Chandra Shekhar Gupta, "Gender Differences in Stress Response: Role of Developmental and Biological Determinants," *Industrial Psychiatry Journal* 20, no. 1 (2011): 4–10. doi: 10.4103/0972-6748.98407.

7. Suzanne B. Feinstein, PhD, and Brian A. Fallon, MD, MPH, "Don't Be Fooled by Hypochondria," *Current Psychiatry* 2, no. 9 (2003): 27–39, https://www.mdedge.com/psychiatry/article/59754/anxiety-disorders/dont-be-fooled-hypochondria.

8. Mathias Wullum Nielsen et al., "One and a Half Million Medical Papers Reveal a Link Between Author Gender and Attention to Gender and Sex Analysis," *Nature Human Behaviour* 1 (2017): 791–796, https://www.nature.com/articles/s41562-017-0235-x.

Chapter 6

1. Laura Kiesel, "Women and Pain: Disparities in Experience and Treatment," *Harvard Health Blog*, October 9, 2017, https://www.health.harvard.edu/blog/women-and-pain-disparities-in-experience-and-treatment-2017100912562; Roger B. Fillingim et al., "Sex, Gender, and Pain: A Review of Recent Clinical and Experimental Findings," *Journal of Pain* 10, no. 5 (2009): 447–485. doi: 10.1016/j.jpain.2008.12.001; Bruce Becker, MD, and Alyson J. McGregor, MD, MA, "Article Commentary: Men, Women, and Pain," *Gender and the Genome*, 46–50. https://doi.org/10.1089/gg.2017.0002.

2. Justin L. Hay et al., "Determining Pain Detection and Tolerance Thresholds Using an Integrated, Multi-Modal Pain Task Battery," *Journal of Visualized Experiments* 110 (2016): 53800. doi: 10.3791/53800.

3. Robert E. Sorge and Larissa J. Strath, "Sex Differences in Pain Responses," *Current Opinion in Physiology* 6 (2018): 75–81. doi: 10.1016/j.cophys.2018.05.006.

4. Robert E. Sorge et al., "Different Immune Cells Mediate Mechanical Pain Hypersensitivity in Male and Female Mice," *Nature Neuroscience* 18, no. 8 (2015): 1081–1083. doi: 10.1038/nn.4053.

5. R. Y. North et al., "Electrophysiological and Transcriptomic Correlates of Neuropathic Pain in Human Dorsal Root Ganglion Neurons," *Brain* 142, no. 5 (2019): 1215–1226. doi: 10.1093/brain/awz063.

6. Joel D. Greenspan et al., "Studying Sex and Gender Differences in Pain and Analgesia: A Consensus Report," *Pain* 132, Suppl. 1 (2007): S26–S45. doi: 10.1016/j.pain.2007.10.014.

7. Elena H. Chartoff and Maria Mavrikaki, "Sex Differences in Kappa Opioid Receptor Function and Their Potential Impact on Addiction," *Frontiers in Neuroscience* 9 (2015): 466. doi: 10.3389/fnins.2015.00466.

8. Table 2 in Greenspan et al., "Studying Sex and Gender Differences in Pain and Analgesia."

9. JoAnn V. Pinkerton, MD, Christine J. Guico-Pabia, MD, MBA, and Hugh S. Taylor, MD, "Menstrual Cycle–Related Exacerbation of Disease," *American Journal of Obstetrics and Gynecology* 202, no. 3 (2010): 221–231. doi: 10.1016/j.ajog.2009.07.061.

10. Katy Vincent and Irene Tracey, "Hormones and Their Interaction with the Pain Experience," *Pain Reviews* 2, no. 2 (2008): 20–24. doi: 10.1177/204946370800200206.

11. Bruce Becker, MD, and Alyson J. McGregor, MD, MA, "Article Commentary: Men, Women, and Pain," *Gender and the Genome*, 46–50. https://doi.org/10.1089/gg.2017.0002.

12. Diane E. Hoffmann and Anita J. Tarzian, "The Girl Who Cried Pain: A Bias Against Women in the Treatment of Pain," *Journal of Law, Medicine & Ethics* 29 (2001): 13–27. doi: 10.2139/ssrn.383803; C. Noel Bairey Merz, MD, "The Yentl Syndrome and Gender Inequality in Ischemic HD," *Cardiology Today*, August 2011, https://www.healio.com/cardiology/news/print/cardiology-today/%7B7cff01d6-0b82-4d2e-a3c9-aea61a5c61ad%7D/the-yentl-syndrome-and-gender-inequality-in-ischemic-hd.

13. Joe Fassler, "How Doctors Take Women's Pain Less Seriously," *The Atlantic*, October 15, 2015, https://www.theatlantic.com/health/archive/2015/10/emergency-room-wait-times-sexism/410515.

14. Richard E. Harris et al., "Traditional Chinese Acupuncture and Placebo (Sham) Acupuncture Are Differentiated by Their Effects on μ-Opioid Receptors (MORs)," *NeuroImage* 47, no. 3 (2009): 1077–1085. doi: 10.1016/j.neuroimage.2009.05.083.

Chapter 7

1. Vascular Disease Foundation, "Every Five Minutes Someone Dies from a Blood Clot or Deep Vein Thrombosis," *ScienceDaily*, March 5, 2011, https://www.sciencedaily.com/releases/2011/03/110305105233.htm.

2. Yana Vinogradova, Carol Coupland, and Julia Hippisley-Cox, "Use of Combined Oral Contraceptives and Risk of Venous Thromboembolism: Nested Case-Control Studies Using the QResearch and CPRD Databases," *BMJ* 350 (2015). doi: 10.1136/bmj.h2135.

3. Practice Committee of the American Society for Reproductive Medicine, "Combined Hormonal Contraception and the Risk of Venous Thromboembolism: A Guideline," *Fertility and Sterility* 107, no. 1 (2016): 43–51. doi: 10.1016/j.fertnstert.2016.09.027.

4. Erin Wayman, "Hormone Therapy: A Woman's Dilemma," *Endocrine News*, November 2012, https://endocrinenews.endocrine.org/hormone-therapy-a-womans-dilemma.

5. R. B. Fillingim and R. R. Edwards, "The Association of Hormone Replacement Therapy with Experimental Pain Responses in Postmenopausal Women," *Pain* 92, nos. 1–2 (2001): 229–234. doi: 10.1016/s0304-3959(01)00256-1.

6. Kent D. Stening et al., "Hormonal Replacement Therapy Does Not Affect Self-Estimated Pain or Experimental Pain Responses in Post-Menopausal Women Suffering from Fibromyalgia: A Double-Blind, Randomized, Placebo-Controlled Trial," *Rheumatology* 50, no. 3 (2010): 544–551. doi: 10.1093/rheumatology/keq348.

7. Q. Yu et al., "[Comparison of the effect of fluoxetine combined with hormone replacement therapy (HRT) and single HRT in treating menopausal depression]," *Zhonghua Fu Chan Ke Za Zhi* 39, no. 7 (2004): 461–464, https://www.ncbi.nlm.nih.gov/pubmed/15347469.

8. Tam L. Westlund and B. L. Parry, "Does Estrogen Enhance the Antidepressant Effects of Fluoxetine?" *Journal of Affective Disorders* 77, no. 1 (2003): 87–92. doi: 10.1016/s0165-0327(02)00357-9.

9. Talal Alzahrani et al., "Cardiovascular Disease Risk Factors and Myocardial Infarction in the Transgender Population," *Circulation: Cardiovascular*

Quality and Outcomes 12 (2019): e005597. doi.org/10.1161/CIRCOUT
COMES.119.005597; Louis J. Gooren, Katrien Wierckx, and Erik J.
Giltay, "Cardiovascular Disease in Transsexual Persons Treated with
Cross-Sex Hormones: Reversal of the Traditional Sex Difference in Car-
diovascular Disease Pattern," *European Journal of Endocrinology* 170, no. 6
(2014): 809–819. doi: https://doi.org/10.1530/EJE-14-0011.

10. Sarah M. Burke et al., "Testosterone Effects on the Brain in Transgender Men," *Cerebral Cortex* 28, no. 5 (2018): 1582–1596, https://doi
.org/10.1093/cercor/bhx054.

11. Hilleke E. Hulshoff Pol et al., "Changing Your Sex Changes Your Brain:
Influences of Testosterone and Estrogen on Adult Human Brain Structure," *European Journal of Endocrinology* 155 (2006): S107–S114. doi:
10.1530/eje.1.02248.

Chapter 8

1. "Orders Regarding Burial of the Dead Body," al-Islam.org, https://
www.al-islam.org/islamic-laws-ayatullah-abul-qasim-al-khui/orders
-regarding-burial-dead-body.

2. Imam M. Xierali, PhD, and Marc A. Nivet, EdD, MBA, "The Racial and
Ethnic Composition and Distribution of Primary Care Physicians," *Journal of Health Care for the Poor and Underserved* 29, no. 1 (2018): 556–570.
doi: 10.1353/hpu.2018.0036.

3. Audrey Smedley and Brian D. Smedley, "Race as Biology Is Fiction, Rac-
ism as a Social Problem Is Real: Anthropological and Historical Perspec-
tives on the Social Construction of Race," *American Psychologist* 60, no. 1
(2005): 16–26, https://psycnet.apa.org/buy/2005-00117-003.

4. Robert Wood Johnson Foundation, "Reducing Disparities to Improve the
Quality of Care for Racial and Ethnic Minorities," *Quality Field Notes* 4 (2014),
https://www.rwjf.org/en/library/research/2014/06/reducing-disparities
-to-improve-care-for-racial-and-ethnic-minorities.html.

5. Elizabeth Chuck, "How Training Doctors in Implicit Bias Could Save
the Lives of Black Mothers," *NBC News*, May 11, 2018, https://www
.nbcnews.com/news/us-news/how-training-doctors-implicit-bias-could
-save-lives-black-mothers-n873036.

6. American Heart Association, "Racial Disparities Continue for Black Women
Seeking Heart Health Care," *Medical Xpress*, April 5, 2019, https://medicalx
press.com/news/2019-04-racial-disparities-black-women-heart.html.

7. Sandhya Somashekhar, "The Disturbing Reason Some African American Patients May Be Undertreated for Pain," *Washington Post*, April 4, 2016, https://www.washingtonpost.com/news/to-your-health/wp/2016/04/04/do-blacks-feel-less-pain-than-whites-their-doctors-may-think-so; Kelly M. Hoffman et al., "Racial Bias in Pain Assessment and Treatment Recommendations, and False Beliefs About Biological Differences Between Blacks and Whites," *Proceedings of the National Academy of Sciences* (April 4, 2016). doi: 10.1073/pnas.1516047113.

8. Joshua Aronson, PhD, "Unhealthy Interactions: The Role of Stereotype Threat in Health Disparities," *American Journal of Public Health* 103, no. 1 (2013): 50–56. doi: 10.2105/AJPH.2012.300828.

9. "Unequal Treatment: What Healthcare Providers Need to Know About Racial and Ethnic Disparities in Healthcare," *Institute of Medicine: Shaping the Future for Health*, March 2002, https://www.nap.edu/resource/10260/disparities_providers.pdf.

10. William C. Shiel Jr., MD, FACP, FACR, "Medical Definition of Hippocratic Oath," MedicineNet, reviewed on March 6, 2018, https://www.medicinenet.com/script/main/art.asp?articlekey=20909.

11. Laura Castillo-Page, PhD, *Diversity in the Physician Workforce: Facts and Figures 2010* (Washington, DC: Association of American Medical Colleges, 2010), https://www.aamc.org/download/432976/data/factsandfigures2010.pdf.

12. Isobel Bowler, "Ethnic Profile of the Doctors in the United Kingdom: A Diverse Group of Doctors Would Appreciate the Concerns of the Population Better," *BMJ* 329, no. 7466 (2004): 583–584. doi: 10.1136/bmj.329.7466.583; "Number of Registered Doctors in the United Kingdom (U.K.) in 2018, by Gender and Specialty," Statista, https://www.statista.com/statistics/698260/registered-doctors-united-kingdom-uk-by-gender-and-specialty.

13. Nicole Torres, "Research: Having a Black Doctor Led Black Men to Receive More-Effective Care," *Harvard Business Review*, August 10, 2018, https://hbr.org/2018/08/research-having-a-black-doctor-led-black-men-to-receive-more-effective-care.

14. Somnath Saha, MD, MPH, "Student Body Racial and Ethnic Composition and Diversity-Related Outcomes in U.S. Medical Schools," *JAMA* 300, no. 10 (2008): 1135–1145. doi:10.1001/jama.300.10.1135.

15. Brad N. Greenwood, Seth Carnahan, and Laura Huang, "Patient-Physician Gender Concordance and Increased Mortality Among Female

Heart Attack Patients," *PNAS* 115, no. 34 (2018): 8569–8574. doi: 10.1073/pnas.1800097115.

16. Raynard Kington, Diana Tisnado, and David M. Carlisle, "Increasing Racial and Ethnic Diversity Among Physicians: An Intervention to Address Health Disparities?," in *The Right Thing to Do, the Smart Thing to Do: Enhancing Diversity in the Health Professions: Summary of the Symposium on Diversity in Health Professions in Honor of Herbert W. Nickens, M.D.*, ed. B. D. Smedley et al. (Washington, DC: National Academies Press, 2001).

17. Holly Mead et al., *Racial and Ethnic Disparities in U.S. Health Care: A Chartbook* (Washington, DC: Commonwealth Fund, 2008), 95, https://www.commonwealthfund.org/sites/default/files/documents/___media_files_publications_chartbook_2008_mar_racial_and_ethnic_disparities_in_u_s__health_care__a_chartbook_mead_racialethnicdisparities_chartbook_1111_pdf.pdf.

18. M. L. Martin et al., eds., *Diversity and Inclusion in Quality Patient Care* (New York: Springer International Publishing, 2016). doi: 10.1007/978-3-319-22840-2.

19. Jordan J. Cohen, Barbara A. Gabriel, and Charles Terrell, "The Case for Diversity in the Health Care Workforce," *Health Affairs* 21, no. 5 (September/October 2002). doi: 10.1377/hlthaff.21.5.90.

20. C. Puchalski and A. L. Romer, "Taking a Spiritual History Allows Clinicians to Understand Patients More Fully," *Journal of Palliative Medicine* 3, no. 1 (2000): 129–137. doi: 10.1089/jpm.2000.3.129.

Chapter 9

1. M. B. Streiff et al., "Lessons from the Johns Hopkins Multi-disciplinary Venous Thromboembolism (VTE) Prevention Collaborative," *BMJ* 344 (2012): e3935. doi: 10.1136/bmj.e3935.

Chapter 10

1. American Well, "JeffConnect Puts Patients Face-to-Face with Their Doctor over Video," *PR Newswire*, April 10, 2015, https://www.prnewswire.com/news-releases/jeffconnect-puts-patients-face-to-face-with-their-doctor-over-video-300063915.html.

INDEX

Index

Index

Index

Index

Index

Index

ABOUT THE AUTHOR

ALYSON J. McGREGOR, MD, MA, FACEP, is a women's health pioneer who has brought the concept of sex and gender differences in the delivery of acute medical care to the national stage.

She is associate professor of emergency medicine at the Warren Alpert Medical School of Brown University and cofounder and director of the Division of Sex and Gender in Emergency Medicine at Brown University's Department of Emergency Medicine. Dr. McGregor is also cofounder of the Sex and Gender Women's Health Collaborative.

Dr. McGregor's research focus is on the effects of sex and gender on emergent conditions. She has been an advocate for this model nationally, speaking widely to both medical professionals and laypeople. Her TEDx talk, "Why Medicine Often Has Dangerous Side Effects for Women," currently has over 1.5 million views and has sparked a national conversation around how sex and gender influence medical treatment and outcomes.

She has written or cowritten over seventy peer-reviewed publications in scientific journals on the topic of sex and gender. She is also lead editor of the medical textbook *Sex and Gender in Acute Care Medicine*. *Sex Matters* is her first book for the general public.